BEAT HEART DISEASE WITHOUT SURGERY

BEAT HEART DISEASE WITHOUT SURGERY

A consumers' guide to circulation therapy

Jillie Collings

Thorsons
An Imprint of HarperCollins*Publishers*

Thorsons
An Imprint of HarperCollins*Publishers*
77–85 Fulham Palace Road,
Hammersmith, London W6 8JB
1160 Battery Street,
San Francisco, California 94111–1213

Published by Thorsons 1995
1 3 5 7 9 10 8 6 4 2

A catalogue record for this book is available
from the British Library

ISBN 0 7225 3026 9

Printed in Great Britain by
HarperCollinsManufacturing Glasgow

CONTENTS

FOREWORD

WHEN Jillie Collings approached me for the first time to discuss EDTA chelation therapy, my first thought was, '... again?'.

In the many years during which I have practised chelation therapy, various people have sought my assistance or judgement to produce books and articles on the subject. Unfortunately, many of the results contributed little to a better understanding of this treatment. On the contrary, in many cases more questions were created than asked.

After a few minutes listening to Jillie Collings, however, I began to realize that this time it was a different story and that I might be learning a thing or two from her. She knows how to awaken and maintain interest in a subject by letting you know that she is personally involved.

Her book deals with all aspects of chelation therapy – scientific as well as emotional – and is an intriguing read. The scientific part indeed gives a substantiated explanation of the many actions of EDTA and settles with its unsubstantiated reputation as a detergent of blood vessels. It also makes clear that the effect of EDTA may be enhanced by many other orthomolecular and dietary measures.

Jillie Collings does not evade discussing all the controversies that surround this treatment, and she deals with them in an intelligent and convincing way because her knowledge of the matter is impressive. It is difficult for the layperson to understand that such a simple, effective and harmless treatment meets so much unreasonable opposition from orthodox physicians.

Beat Heart Disease Without Surgery points out very clearly that patients should not assume the classic passive attitude. For optimal results, they should participate actively in the treatment. The book furnishes all the information needed for such an approach. It makes patients aware of the importance of their own contribution in the healing of their ailment.

The administration of EDTA chelation therapy cannot be stopped any longer, despite attempts from orthodox medicine. It is probably one of the most consistently increasing unorthodox treatments of atherosclerotic cardiovascular disease. The training and testing of physicians in this therapy is well organized and is conducted by the American College for Advancement in Medicine and the American Board of Chelation Therapy. An international board is expected to be instituted in 1995.

Jillie Collings's book is an important contribution to better understanding of EDTA chelation therapy and related orthomolecular medicine.* I feel privileged to introduce it to you.

Peter J. Van Der Schaar MD, Ph.D.
Vice-chairman of the International
Board of Chelation Therapy

---

* Nobel prize-winning scientist Linus Pauling describes orthomolecular medicine as 'the preservation of good health and the treatment of disease by varying the concentrations in the human body of substances that are normally present in the body and are required for health'.

INTRODUCTION

THERE is no longer any doubt that contemporary orthodox treatments for heart disease, such as bypass surgery and angioplasty, and to a certain extent drug therapy, are failing to address the problem. At most, they are giving a stay of execution from what is a life-threatening disease, but they are not effecting a cure.

Orthodox medicine has become perfectly aware of this through the perusal of certain landmark scientific trials which have taken place over the past 20 years on both sides of the Atlantic. These have shown conclusively that unless patients are suffering from a particularly severe form of coronary artery (heart) disease, such as an obstruction in the left main coronary artery or what is known as triple coronary vessel disease, which only 10 per cent do, the rest live longer if they do not have surgery.

The trials show that alternative treatment by drugs is preferable to surgery. But are drugs the only alternative? What is well-known to both patient and doctor is that drugs are not effecting a cure any more than surgery; they are simply controlling a potentially dangerous health condition, rather like sentries posted at the sites of potential sources of uprising. And drugs take their toll because nearly all of them have side effects of one kind or another – some of them severe. Furthermore, when one is put on drugs it is very difficult (though not impossible) to quit, as whatever symptoms were being experienced worsen considerably for a time. And inevitably, as the condition which is merely being suppressed by the drugs slowly worsens, surgery may become the only option left.

What is the bewildered patient to do when faced with a potentially lethal disease, the orthodox treatment options for which are rather like choosing between the devil and the deep blue sea? Surely there are other options to surgery and drug therapy?

There are. And it is something of a scandal that the general public have so little knowledge of one treatment in particular which is both safe, effective, painless, proven, easy to receive and which definitely reverses the process of arterial clogging, the main cause of heart and other diseases of the circulation.

Called chelation therapy (pronounced key-lay'-shun), it is not new, it is not untested and it is definitely not to be overlooked by anyone with heart or arterial disease, because once the disease has become established to the point where there are diagnosable symptoms, some kind of interventive therapy is usually needed in order to restore the body to a stage where it can keep up once more with its own repair work.

This book catalogues many other ways in which circulatory problems can be tackled naturally and kept at bay, even reversed, such as with diet, body cleansing techniques, stress management, easy but effective exercise routines, therapeutic nutritional approaches, the use of herbs and one exciting new treatment thought to be a valuable adjunct to chelation therapy – oxygen therapy. But none of these (with the possible exception of oxygen therapy in some cases) are likely to reverse the on-going process of established circulatory disease.

Tremendous improvements are being made now by dietary and nutritional approaches alone, especially in respect to those with moderate or early heart disease – should they be lucky enough to know about it. Regrettably heart disease is usually silent until well-advanced (*see Chapter 1*) – which is why 25 per cent of all first heart-attacks are fatal. Thus it makes sense to get into the habit of having regular checkups both of blood pressure and of blood itself – especially if heart disease runs in your family – before any symptoms appear. It may be too late otherwise.

Prevention is the fundament of modern health practice and stands every person in good stead, because moderate changes in one's diet and lifestyle implemented in one's thirties or forties or even earlier, can usually control whatever is the incipient problem. Chapters 1, 2 and 4 tell you about risk factors and how to get such checks done and how to follow them up.

If this principle is followed, the need for strong intervention, which always carries some element of risk for the body, only has to occur when we have been consciously or unconsciously making hay while the sun shines for far too long. The body is a self-healing system, given half a chance.

Fortunately our understanding of how the body works, ages and becomes susceptible to degenerative diseases, such as heart disease, arthritis and cancer, has progressed by leaps and bounds in the last few decades. A revolution is going on in health care and the essential ingredient of this revolution is that maintaining good health comes down to each individual following a lifetime plan of prevention/protection, involving a healthy diet and lifestyle patterns accompanied by an awareness of what constitutes their own health risk, taking into account family weaknesses, environmental and occupational pressures and sundry relationships.

But why aren't we being counselled about this by our local GPs? Many of them are performing heroic efforts in trying to teach their patients about changing negative diet and lifestyle patterns before it is too late. But in certain ways GPs are constricted from passing on information about new therapies and lines of thought if these have not yet been officially recognized by the medical establishment which governs them all.

Regrettably there are signs that where some of these new innovative therapies threaten a vast number of medical lifestyles and practices, they are being adopted extremely slowly. Chapter 8 investigates evidence of the stranglehold which vested interests (such as the drug companies) may have on medical policy-making.

Whilst we may like to believe that any therapy involving such vast numbers of the general public as are concerned in treatments for the circulation must stem from the basic rule of healing 'first do no harm', it seems otherwise when we examine some statistics (such as those to do with the long-term efficacy of angioplasty and bypass surgery – *see Chapter 3*).

Indeed it would seem that we (the public) are the innocent victims of some kind of power struggle which is taking place over who controls health care and the many billions of revenue it represents. We must always remember that bad health generates income; good health generates very little but joy to those who have it.

Being aware of this should make us all the more determined to follow a policy of prevention, and when in need of treatment to be a little suspicious of every option which is suggested to us, be it orthodox or alternative, until we have researched it, read about it, spoken to people who have had it and assessed those who offer it. Then and only then can we hope to find the best way to tackle our individual heart (or other) problem.

A PERSONAL INTRODUCTION TO CHELATION THERAPY AND OTHER MEASURES FOR THE CIRCULATION

I did not know a great deal about arterial/heart disease (typical of those who have it and don't realize it) until a colleague suggested that I write about a brilliant alternative therapy for clearing the entire circulatory system (including the coronary arteries) in the alternative health column I was then writing for the British newspaper the *Guardian*.

It was 1988 and the first clinic to practise this technique had opened in London in 1985. My colleague's own father had been helped greatly by chelation, having been given up as too great a risk for surgery by the medical profession.

My colleague proposed that there might be many other people in a similar situation to his father, to say nothing of the many others diagnosed daily as having heart disease. He felt that I was morally bound to tackle this serious health problem, from which Britain has one of the highest death rates in the world – 500 a day – in order to acquaint the public with an alternative to surgery and drug therapy, since those were not affecting a cure.

I was not so easily convinced: I was choosing my subjects very carefully in order to build what I thought was a necessary bridge between alternative and orthodox health approaches and hence tended to steer clear of concepts which seemed too radical or controversial. In a way I was behaving like the establishment of alternative health, but I was soon to be relieved of this attitude by what, upon preparatory investigation, I began to see was a valuable therapeutic adjunct to the treatment of arterial disease, one which was being unaccountably ignored by medicine, even though it is traditionally practised under the orthodox umbrella by doctors of medicine. In fact some of the early evidence I

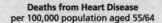

Deaths from Heart Disease
per 100,000 population aged 55/64

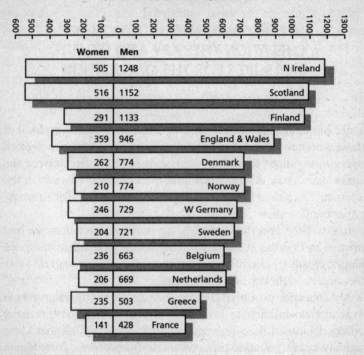

Women	Men	
505	1248	N Ireland
516	1152	Scotland
291	1133	Finland
359	946	England & Wales
262	774	Denmark
210	774	Norway
246	729	W Germany
204	721	Sweden
236	663	Belgium
206	669	Netherlands
235	503	Greece
141	428	France

examined pointed to its being suppressed*.

It is said that every research writer in the course of their career lands an issue which won't leave them alone: chelation therapy, or to cast the net slightly wider, therapies for cleansing and rejuvenating the body such as ozone therapy, and the much misunderstood therapies for cleansing the colon, such as colonic irrigation (or hydrotherapy to give it its modern name) have become mine.

After obsessively careful research, I wrote my first article about Chelation Therapy in 1988 for the *Guardian* and over one thousand readers responded. Many of these went on to have the therapy and, seven years later, are represented by two of the four case histories I present in this book (*see Chapter 8*).

*James P. Cater MD, PhD, *Racketeering in Medicine: The Suppression of Alternatives*, Hampton Roads, USA, 1992. *Also see Chapter 8*.

Part of my research included my decision to undergo, guinea-pig fashion, the painless diagnostic technique (using echolocation sound waves much like sonar used by submarines) deployed by the clinic to check my own arterial disease status. To my (and their) horror I discovered that some of my arteries were significantly blocked, the most serious (to me) being the right carotid artery which was nearly 50 per cent obstructed. (The clinic insisted that their diagnosis be independently checked, which it was at Guy's Hospital who confirmed the original readings.)

The internal carotid is the chief artery leading to the brain which passes close to the ear. This diagnosis explained some rather vague symptoms which I had been putting down to pressure of work and an old ear abscess, like tinnitus – ringing in the ear – (it was a new symptom so I don't know why I blamed it on the old ear abscess), as well as increasing tiredness of the eyes despite stronger glasses and difficulty in concentrating after a certain period in the day, when I had been accustomed to being able to read and study well into the night.

I had the treatment (a course of 17 chelations) and was greatly helped by it and subsequent tests have confirmed that my arteries have opened and have become more bouncy and resilient. A factor of arterial disease is hardening of arterial walls and it is this and the narrowing of their bore that are the vital factors in the causation of high blood pressure, since the heart is trying to push blood through increasingly furred-up pipes which have also lost much of their rubbery ability to expand with the pulse. This makes the heart work all that much harder, setting up a vicious circle of slow but inevitable debilitation – unless of course, in my lucky case, treatment intervenes in time.

Since having the initial 17 treatments (and later eight more making 25 in all), I have continued to improve. My level of mental alertness has reverted to what it used to be and vague symptoms of pain in the feet and calf muscles have disappeared completely (this I had been attributing to an old back injury – it is amazing how we can fool ourselves about symptoms).

I have also changed my diet to include less meat and more oily fish, considerably less dairy products and more vegetables, fruit and cereals. And I now take fish oil supplements, oat bran, lecithin, plenty of vitamins A, C and E and a variety of protective minerals.*

Last year I had my first course of oxygen (ozone) therapy which also had a dramatically helpful effect; this time on energy and vitality. Lately I have been working six and seven days a week, sometimes for eight or nine hours, on this book because I want to spend some time with my grown-up son of 33 when he arrives later this summer from Australia. This is one mature guinea pig who is not going to die, but rather benefit from her experiments. Hopefully my years of careful research into heart-lifting therapies and measures will help others too.

---

*Fortunately, I did not have to cut down on sugar, or any products made from it, which is the prime dietary requirement for the control of heart disease (*see Chapter 7*) as I ate very little of it or of refined foods made with white flour, etc.

CHAPTER ONE

UNDERSTANDING HEART DISEASE AND AGEING

L ET's settle one issue right from the start: heart disease is wrongly named. Heart disease is really arterial or circulatory disease, but the term 'heart' is so widely used and understood that even the medical profession continue to use it. Whatever the term used, the disease covers a wide spectrum of complaints, including:

- angina (chest pain on exertion or stressful experience)
- intermittent claudication (pains or cramps in the leg on walking or hurrying)
- dizziness, throbbing or tightness in the head
- confusion, difficulty in concentrating
- increasing breathlessness on exertion
- increasing coldness, weakness or heaviness of the extremities
- general feelings of tension, throbbing or fullness when under pressure
- ringing in the ears (tinnitus), problems with vision or hearing
- swelling of the ankles, unrelated to injury or other causes
- high blood pressure (this last is usually diagnosed by a doctor as a result of symptoms such as those described above)

These symptoms are very varied, but it is hardly surprising that the signs of arterial disease are numerous and indefinite when it is considered that the human body contains no less than 30,000 *miles* of arteries – some estimates put it even higher. These traverse every square inch of the body, and comprise the network through which vital blood circulates to the tissues. Thus, there is a wide variety of sites which can be affected and in different ways, depending on individual lifestyles and hereditary factors.

It is no statistical secret, however, that in contemporary times the heart (through disease of its coronary artery system) is most frequently affected, as is revealed by the high incidence of heart attacks in our society. In 1991 in Britain, they accounted for a quarter of all deaths; the figure in America corresponds. Coming a close second to heart incidents are those which relate to the head (of which strokes are the most serious) and the legs (intermittent

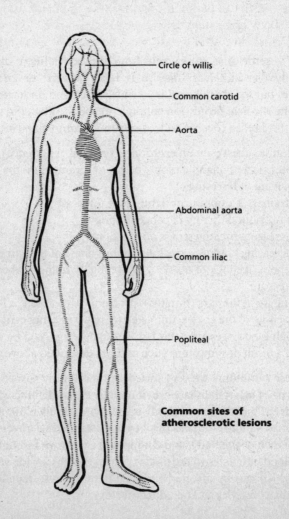

Common sites of atherosclerotic lesions

claudication), causing circulatory difficulties which are so severe in some cases that amputation has to be considered. Computing these into the mortality rates reveals that by far the largest number of deaths in the western world are due to arterial causes.

Arterial diseases are progressive and serious, because they adversely affect the conveyance of vital supplies of oxygen and nutrients to body tissues. They also prejudice the removal of waste products which can poison the tissues if they build up sufficiently. Since all body organs and their functions depend on blood circulation for their successful operation, it can be seen just how widespread the effects of arterial disease can be. Yet their effects are largely silent until arteries become 90 per cent blocked, which is why some 25 per cent of first heart attacks occur without warning. Somehow enough blood manages to squeeze through until then to keep us relatively free of symptoms. Whether this is a good thing or a bad is questionable. The body's main aim seems to be to keep the show on the road for as long as possible. But when it finally does give in the symptoms are usually serious, as statistics once more confirm.

Strokes, too, can occur without warning. In one second they can change the life of a seemingly healthy individual into that of a frightened invalid, in some cases even ending it. There seems to be no rhyme or reason, let alone justice, in such sudden transformations. But in fact there will have been plenty of minor warnings, even major ones, were we to be wise to the symptoms and to keep a closer watching brief on the body that is in our care. Many a man has complained of pains in his left arm radiating into the neck before he drops with a heart attack, and this is a classic sign that a heart checkup is needed. Many a person has attributed worsening pains in the legs and feet to an old back injury, or the weather, when in fact they may be the signs of increasingly blocked leg arteries.

Since such conditions are likely to affect the health of one in three of us severely, and all of us to a certain extent (because good health depends on good blood circulation), it is as well to consider:

a) what preventive measures can be taken to avoid serious
   arterial disease and,

b) what treatment options are available should an emergency arise.

Imagine the scenario of a wife who has heard that her husband has had a heart attack at work and is now in intensive care and is being advised that he needs a coronary bypass operation. Does she have any choice but to agree? Can she even choose who does this major surgery? Or decide which hospital? And all the while her husband, with whom she is used to consulting, lies helpless requiring her to make decisions at the worst possible time – in an emergency. No wonder such decisions are often left to the experts: it is too late to examine what alternatives there may have been or what precautions may have been taken to avoid such a scenario.

Wealth v. Health

In matters of wealth it is accepted practice in society to make decisions early: to take advice from several, often opposing, sources of information and then to make financial decisions which are quite independent of either. It is also accepted practice to make provisions for the future, and to update one's financial picture on a regular basis.

In matters of health it seems that a whole different ball game exists, one that leaves the individual very little choice or say in matters that are directly connected to life itself and the preservation of it. In one area it is generally thought that it would be foolish to trust blindly, in another, it would seem that total trust is the order of the day.

Yet there are increasing signs that health and wealth are inextricably connected. They have to be, because modern health care has become a very expensive business. Awareness of this need not make us suspicious, but it should make us more cautious, more aware of our options.

Then too, the changing face of health care and the speed at which current health knowledge and techniques are being superseded, means that no establishment, however worthy, can incorporate them into its structure quickly enough. It is both the strength and weakness of establishments, such as the medical establishment, that they are cautious in adopting new procedures. (We will go into this in more detail in Chapter 8 when we examine how cautious they are in adopting new surgical procedures universally without recourse to clinical trials and studies to test their efficacy first. But for now we are looking at whether the practice of placing your health blindly in their hands for them to make decisions about it at some future date is wise, especially considering the times in which we live.

The Changing Face of Health Care

There is a revolution going on in health and new information is coming up thick and fast. It is information which will ultimately change the whole face of health care. To give a practical example of the magnitude of this change, it is being confidently posited by health scientists on the frontiers that vitamins and vitamin therapy will largely take over from drugs and be our new 'medicine'. (NB: In America sales of vitamins to the public have been controlled since 1993. One can only assume that in the face of overwhelming evidence which has been gathering for two or three decades that health authorities are sensing where the new wealth in health will be and are stepping in to control it. There are attempts to do likewise in the European Union.)

Another acknowledged health trend for the future is the adoption of prevention as an active principle in health care (i.e. a stitch in time saves nine) rather than the intervention (last ditch) system we have now. In terms of heart and arterial health this may mean starting much earlier than was previously thought to be necessary if we are to reverse this socially destructive trend.

In his new book, *A Doctor in the Wilderness*, GP of 30 years' experience, Walter Yellowlees, writes of information which came to light as long ago as 1951, when the disturbing findings of post mortem examinations of American soldiers killed in Korea showed extensive evidence of advanced coronary artery disease in 77 per cent of cases who were aged on average 22 years.

When it is remembered that arterial disease can remain undiscovered until arteries are up to 90 per cent blocked this is more easily understood, but does this state of affairs have to be? Must we wait until bypass surgery, angioplasty (all described in Chapter 3) and other interventive surgical measures, themselves carrying a significant element of risk, can offer us only a small extension of life, a stay of execution?

Arteriosclerosis: Twentieth Century Disease

Another question which needs to be addressed is: why was coronary artery (heart) disease and in fact all arterial disease virtually unknown until well into this century? Diagnostic and post mortem techniques were not so primitive that they could not assess the cause of death in most cases.

Evidence mounts that the answer lies at the door of modern (i.e. post World War II) diet and lifestyle. Fast foods, a high intake of animal and dairy fats and worse, artificially produced dairy substitutes, plus the huge increase in sugar consumption and in canned, packaged and processed foods (with their high salt content and cocktail of chemical preservatives) are all contributory. Our sedentary, often high pressure lifestyles and modern industrial pollution add two final straws. Chapter 6 presents all this evidence and some very heartening remedies so that our children need never suffer so.

But what of the vast tracts of population caught between the pages of the revolution? We may have dropped, through no real fault of our own, six, seven or eight of our nine stitches and may not have much time, arterially speaking, to undo what we have smoked, eaten, drunk and breathed for several decades. Are we doomed to have radical surgery one day on the one or two inches of arteries serving the vital organs of the heart, brain or legs – reconstructing them by bypass surgery techniques or blasting them open by angioplasty while there remain some 29,999.999 miles of arteries in similar poor shape? Surely this would equate with putting a good patch on the worst puncture of a perished rubber tyre. In fact the analogy is a particularly good one, because rubber perishes in a process not unlike that which happens to the artery walls as we age – and indeed to all other tissues in the body.

Turning Back the Age-Clock

Arresting this ageing process of the tissues at a cellular level is the key to controlling all degenerative diseases, such as cancer, arthritis, Alzheimer's, and in particular the ubiquitous one of arterial disease or atherosclerosis. Like cancer which has metastasized, arterial disease when it is present is all-pervasive. In fact some modern scientists liken the cell proliferation which occurs within the arteries to a form of cancer, since the cells there are multiplying out of control.

Viewed in this light it can be seen how pointless surgical intervention is, except as a life-saving measure at key sites such as the heart. (And even then recent statistics from America, home of bypass surgery, are revealing that no more than 21 per cent of all bypass operations in America can be considered effective.) Yet current attitudes within the medical establishment reveal that their solution to the appalling increase in arterially-related diseases is not to consider rejuvenating therapies such as the one advocated in this book, that is oral and intravenous chelation therapy, but to train more heart surgeons! That's official (*see Chapter 8*).

The Smallest Common Denominator of Disease: The Cell

To understand what's going on, or wrong in contemporary bodies one has to go to the smallest common denominator in the body, the cell. There are some 60-75 trillion of these in the average body, and the health of each individual depends on how well those individual cells are functioning.

Each one is a living chemical factory, a miraculous and precise production unit which uses nutrients from food and oxygen from breathing in order to produce energy, the energy for life. Each one is interconnected and at an unconscious level the brain is aware of what is going on in all of them. (That could be one big reason why nine tenths of the brain seem not to be concerned with our conscious lives.)

Scientists have known about the cells and how they work for a number of years, but until recently they have not understood fully what goes wrong when a cell goes out of control and proliferates, such as with cancer, or malfunctions, as with Alzheimer's, or clogs up with cholesterol and calcium, as with atherosclerosis.

One thing is becoming clear, though, and that is that any treat-

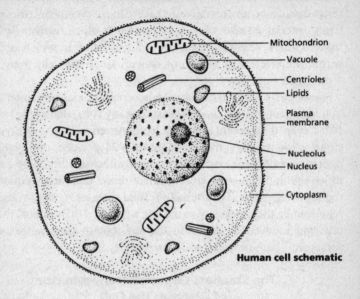

Human cell schematic

ment for any of the above degenerative diseases will have to work at a cellular (molecular) level to be effective in redressing them.

It is curious that significant biological advances seem to happen in quantum leaps (although in fact they are being worked on constantly – it is their acceptance which takes the time), and the era we are in now corresponds to that of about 100 years ago when scientists finally learned what happens to the body when cell activity becomes distorted by external infections and, as a result, the germ theory was born. This understanding led to huge advances being made in the control of *infectious* diseases.

A few decades ago, a leap of corresponding importance was achieved in respect of understanding the cause of cell malfunction in *degenerative* diseases and the *free radical theory* was born. It is this which has explained arterial or circulatory disease and it is this, and the application of its understanding, which will ultimately help check ageing – not cure it, but check it. One of its chief indicators is, of course, the onset of arterial disease.

The Free Radical Factor in Ageing and Arterial Disease

According to scientists such as Dr Denham Harmon, formulator of the free radical theory of ageing, and Dr Yuki Niwa, key researcher into substances which combat it, we should live to the age of 100 or 120. The fact that we do not is due to an internal destructive process which takes place at cellular level in the body (and in particular in the arteries where the constant movement of blood accelerates biological activity) called free radical damage.

To understand this phenomenon, it helps to recall the common illustration of an atom with a number of electrons revolving about it in a series of concentric rings – simplistically a bit like the appearance of the planet Saturn and its moons. The electrons in orbit around such atoms are normally paired in order to balance each other's magnetic moments and thus create stability.

However if a pair of electrons gets separated, an unbalanced situation results and the unpaired electron goes on a combining frenzy. Molecules containing these uncoupled electrons are very reactive and destructive and are known as free radicals. In order to satisfy

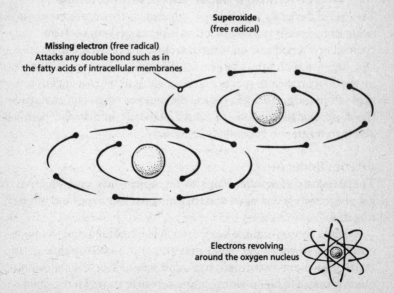

Superoxide
(free radical)

Missing electron (free radical)
Attacks any double bond such as in
the fatty acids of intracellular membranes

Electrons revolving
around the oxygen nucleus

their electrical need they can steal electrons from stable molecules, which in turn steal from others thus creating a chain reaction of tissue destruction.

Although the life of each free radical can only be measured in fractions of milliseconds, millions of them can be created in a moment of stress or by a chemical event or infection in the body, resulting in local cell destruction and thus infinitesimally disrupting the life processes.

Enough of these events occurring in the course of life will eventually become significant. This is not helped by modern lifestyles which have transpired to herd us all together into environments which, for one reason or another, promote further free radical activity – for which read ageing.

To balance this picture, it should be said that free radical activity occurs naturally in the body as well, such as during the metabolic breakdown of organic compounds. Free radical activity is actually deployed by the immune system to zap foreign invaders such as bacteria, so under controlled conditions it does have its uses.

Free Radical Disease and Arterial Damage

Because of the location of arteries, adjacent as they are to the circulation of turbulent rushing blood as it bears oxygen, nutrients and chemicals, wanted and unwanted, around the body, it can be seen why they are such prime targets for this kind of damage. The ultimate effect on their tissues is much the same as when a cut apple is exposed to the air (oxygen radical damage) or when fats go rancid (lipid peroxidation) both of which activities impair the body's ability to repair and rehabilitate its tissues.

Arteries Under Attack

The structure of arteries helps to reveal just how and why they get progressively damaged and then clogged by repair (and other) material.

Arteries consist of three layers, much like a garden hose: a tough outer layer to withstand blood pressure, a muscular middle layer which allows for expansion and contraction with the pulse and helps propel the blood along, and a sensitive inner lining. Unlike garden hoses, arteries are living organisms, producing enzymes and other protective substances to combat free radical damage.

Unfortunately, this protective enzyme process slows down as we age and as factors such as tobacco smoke, pollutants, organic solvents, pesticides, food additives, and heavy metals enter our systems. Dietary imbalances contribute too by creating a raw defence material shortfall. As a result the inner arterial layer, or endothelium, becomes especially vulnerable to minute scarring from free radicals and molecules of heavy metals such as lead, which is a prime destroyer of one of the body's major protective enzymes, glutathione peroxidase.

As tiny graze-like injuries appear in the arterial wall, platelets from the blood rush in to try and stop any bleeding and repair the damage (this is the blood clotting phenomenon without which we would die when we cut ourselves). Unfortunately, the aggregation of platelets cause clumps to form and these attract globules of fat (so prevalent in the western diet) and ultimately bits of calcium (also prevalent in western diets) which together form a kind of plaque just like that which builds up on teeth.

These hardened deposits compromise healthy cell activity further and scientists now think that the irritation actually causes cells to proliferate and go out of control just like cancer cells. The hardened and narrowed arteries force the heart to work harder to pump blood (enter the high blood pressure factor) and the protrusions which jut out into the bloodstream create an additional factor – turbulence in blood flow.

Under this swirling influence bits of plaque can break off and clog smaller vessels, which in key spots like the brain or heart can instigate strokes or heart attacks caused by starvation of blood (ischaemia) to the tissues beyond the blockage. Since the coronary arteries feeding the heart muscle are no more than the size of matchsticks, it is easy to see how and why these are so easily clogged. When they become totally blocked, part of the heart muscle ceases to function, causing a muscle spasm much like cramp (angina) or if extensive enough, a full-scale heart attack.

Enter the heart surgeon to perform crisis surgery and ano ther person steps out on the rocky road, not to cure and recovery,

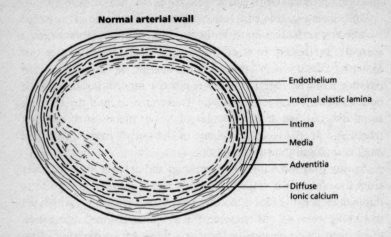

Early atherosclerotic plaque showing a comparatively small amount of diffuse ionic calcium. At this early stage no calcium apatite is evident.

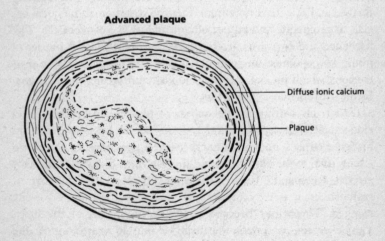

Advanced atherosclerotic plaque showing the build-up of ionic calcium and calcium apatite (plaque).

but to a series of surgical (stop-gap) measures to repair his or her main pump. If the occlusion affects the brain instead of the heart, operations are rarely feasible because of the damage caused by them.

Why is this happening when there are many ways of combating the damage caused by free radicals other than by trying to cut or bore out its results? That, says Paracelsus, is like trying to cure winter by brushing away snow (*see Chapter 7*). Research done by leading heart disease guru, Dr Dean Ornish, and nobel-prize winner, Linus Pauling (*see Chapters 6 and 7*), have established that diet, exercise and anti-stress measures are often all that is needed to arrest the progress of heart disease. Moreover, because they operate on the whole body and take effect at cellular level they are not just stemming the tide of the disease, but turning it around.

In subsequent chapters research concerning diet, exercise and stress-control will be presented and programmes discussed. However, it is sometimes necessary to take more immediate measures than those of diet, exercise and stress-control. When a disease has been in progress for several decades, it may require a stronger interventive step to re-create balance (homeostasis) in the body, after which other, more natural measures can preserve the status quo.

Introducing Circulation Therapy

As I mentioned before, circulation diseases can be very advanced before they are discovered. In such cases therapeutic intervention may be needed and the obvious one, the one which is destined to become the base from which all other measures can stem, is revolutionary, safe and effective chelation therapy.

Overwhelming evidence shows that this, followed by a sensible regime of exercise, diet and relaxation can disperse even advanced arterial plaque and free up the entire arterial system.

Aims of Circulation Therapy, including Chelation

There are many options to consider in the treatment of this complex disease, of which for a small percentage, the surgical option is not to be discounted. This should be viewed, however, according to the opinions of chelating physicians, from a completely different point of value. Instead of its being used as an early option, it should be used as the last in a line of options. To quote the words of Dr Wayne Perry, Medical Director of the Arterial Disease Clinic in London. 'Surgery is becoming more and more aggressive and happening sooner and sooner. You're also getting younger and younger people with less advanced arterial disease having it. Of course the results are going to be better but what of the long-term picture? They will only be faced with further operations in the future.' *(See Chapters 3 and 7 about long-term effectiveness of angioplasty, etc.)*

Dr Perry joins major chelating physicians in eliciting what is a consensus of modern values to be considered when selecting a programme of circulation therapy:

- Safety
- Facility to improve the quality of life long-term
- Reduction of symptoms
- Reduction of drug therapy and supportive medication
- Prevention of the surgical option

Given these values, the basis of new thought in beating existing heart and circulatory disease is:

- A course of chelation therapy
- Supportive (and complementary) oxygen therapy
- Diet and nutritional measures
- Appropriate exercise routines
- Lifestyle/relaxation adaptations as may be necessary

Some people may only need one or two of these measures: others, many of whom may have had surgery or be contemplating it, may need regular maintenance with a therapy such as chelation and regular health maintenance programmes. It all depends on the stage of the disease and other risk factors, such as where a person lives, what they do for a living, how stressful their life is, etc. You can judge your risk factor by reading the ensuing list and processing the diagrammatic form.

Risk Factors in Circulatory (Heart) Disease

Dr Wayne Perry, in material prepared for the Royal College of General Practitioners' Official Reference Book, gave the following general factors as those characteristically predisposing the individual to atherosclerosis: *'male sex, age, hypertension, diabetes, smoking, a family history of premature arterial disease, certain rare metabolic defects such as homocystinuria, and – though this is more controversial – lack of exercise and mental stress.'*

Now ask yourself the following questions (to assess more specific risk factors):

- ❥ Do you eat a lot of fat and dairy products?
- ❥ Do you love, and frequently eat, salty and sweet things?
- ❥ Do you drink coffee regularly and strong tea?
- ❥ Do you have more than three alcoholic drinks daily?
- ❥ Do you eat meat or animal products including eggs more than once a day?
- ❥ Do you eat a lot of canned and processed foods?
- ❥ Do you live in a polluted area?
- ❥ Do you smoke?
- ❥ Are you overweight?
- ❥ Do you have a stressful job/lifestyle?
- ❥ Are you over 30?

If you answer at least half of these questions in the affirmative (particularly the last four), then you may already have circulatory disease and be a candidate for oral or intravenous chelation. And it may be wise for you to have your arteries checked (which can be done by a safe, non-invasive and inexpensive test (*see chapter 4*) after which you can take restorative action, either through diet and lifestyle changes (*see chapter 6*) or through choosing preventative therapy.

A stitch in time may save nine or more very unpleasant surgical ones.

Risk Factor Analysis for Arterial Disease

Family History	Circle and add points
Coronary disease in a 1st degree relative before the age of 55	3.0
Coronary disease in a 1st degree relative before the age of 65	2.5
Coronary disease in a 2nd degree relative before the age of 65	1.0
Stroke in a 1st degree relative before the age of 55	1.0
Stroke in a 2nd degree relative before the age of 65	0.5

Cholesterol and Triglycerides

Cholesterol greater than 220 mg/dL (7 mmol/L)	2.0
Cholesterol greater than 190 mg/dL (6 mmol/L)	1.0
Triglycerides greater than 220 mg/dL (2.5 mmol/L)	0.5

Other Risks

Smoking regularly	1.5
Diabetes	1.0
No regular exercise	1.0
Blood pressure greater than 140/90	0.5
More than 20% overweight	0.5
Type A behaviour	0.5

Risk Score	Increased Risk
3.0	2 x
3.5	3 x
4.0	5 x
4.5	6 x
5.0	15 x
5.5	Not yet calculable

from Arterial Disease Clinic, UK

CHAPTER TWO

INTRODUCING EDTA CHELATION THERAPY: THE BACKBONE OF CIRCULATION THERAPY

EVERY so often in the history of chemistry a substance arises which appears to have one kind of use and later turns out to have other, multifarious uses. Such a substance was discovered in the mid-nineteenth century, a substance which today is being used to thin the blood of those suffering from constrictions of the coronary arteries and other symptoms of arteriosclerosis. At the time of its discovery, it was never thought to have this facility, it was used for the relief of pain.

The substance was aspirin, naturally derived at that time from the bark of willow. Today there is no patent on aspirin – any drug company can make it, and as a result it is cheap, widely available and provided it is used within accepted dose parameters, quite safe. There is even infant aspirin to demonstrate this fact.

EDTA – Ethylene-Diamene-Tetra-Acetate – the substance used to chelate, that is remove, plaque from arteries, is equally a curiosity – an orphan drug, some call it, in that it too was formulated for a completely different purpose and it too can be made by any drug company because its patent has expired. Which means, of course, that, like aspirin, nobody stands to make excessive profits from it – the natural law of competition would bring those profits down.

This, in a nutshell, is why you may not have heard of chelation therapy as an option for the treatment of arterial disease: not because it is unsafe, or unsuccessful in this context, but because no drug company will spend the billions of dollars needed to prove these criteria by the medically required protocol of double blind trials (the cost of which needs to be recouped later in sales).

This does not alter the fact that literally millions of treatments have been performed successfully, mainly in America, but in

Australia, New Zealand, South America and Europe as well, on hundreds of thousands of people suffering with what is customarily advanced arterial disease (people do not seek unusual solutions until the regular ones have failed). And all without a single death attributable to EDTA (Chelation) therapy where it has been administered correctly. (This proviso is important, since earlier in its history it got a bad name with the medical profession for not being as safe as it is, because it was occasionally used incorrectly in the treatment of lead poisoning (*see pages 33–4 and Chapter 5 for details*).

That said, its origins and history can be contemplated with contemporary understanding, and a fascinating history it is, bound up with politics, wars and specific commercial interests which have little or no bearing on its applications today.

EDTA: The Substance, its Evolution and Application

EDTA is a man-made, but nevertheless 'natural' substance in that it mimics the action of an amino acid. Amino acids, formed from ingested proteins, are the building blocks of the body, each one having a specific and vital function in body chemistry. Some amino acids have the ability to bind metal or mineral ions (tiny sub-particles), facilitating their absorption and mobilization for the purposes of tissue-building, etc.

EDTA both mimics and heightens this function, in that it is able to form stable bonds with (in this case) unwanted metals, such as those contributing to arterial disease, thus facilitating their absorption, transportation, and ultimately excretion from the body. This process is called chelation and copies nature in that it uses one substance (the chelator) to carry another substance, the mineral or metal, throughout the body, either to be utilized or excreted. A working example of this process is found in haemoglobin, an active constituent of red blood cells, which is a chelator (carrier) of iron, another vital constituent of blood.

When the body has an excess of a substance (often due to a faulty diet) it tends to store it in an insoluble form away from the bloodstream where it could interfere with body processes. Arterial plaque, consisting of fatty deposits, fibrous repair tissue and calcium, is a classic example of this. Once it is in position, it is very difficult to shift.

This is where EDTA comes in, because it can be used to mobilize insoluble metal deposits in body tissues, especially those in unwanted sites, such as the calcium which binds arterial plaque. Once this has been mobilized, other components of plaque can be more easily disseminated. It is important to note here that there is overwhelming evidence (*see Chapter 5*) that EDTA does not interfere with calcium where it is correctly situated, such as in the bones and teeth. But it can and does mobilize heavy metals like lead and mercury, as well as calcium, which is a distinct advantage in our polluted times, because there is strong evidence to show that heavy metals actually contribute to arterial disease. They behave as irritants, causing unnatural cell growth in arterial walls, as well as being toxic, thus suppressing valuable protective enzyme activity and energy production in arterial sites.

The EDTA Treatment Mode

The clinical process by which EDTA is used to remove unwanted metals from the body is normally achieved by slowly dripping a solution of it into a vein, after which it travels via the circulation to every square inch of the body cleansing away the plaque. Many of the arteries are tiny, so tiny that only a few red blood cells can squeeze through at a time, but EDTA can reach them.

Even finer are some 10 billion capillary vessels in the network which link arteries (carrying oxygenated blood away from the heart) to veins (carrying it back to be re-oxygenated again). EDTA is able to rejuvenate the entire circulatory system, not just the bits serving vital organs such as the heart, head and legs, as does angioplasty and bypass surgery (*see Chapter 3*).

The whole process takes about four hours, during which time the dose, contained in a plastic container, is hung above the patient who is seated in a comfortable chair. It is not a painful process, not is it unpleasant. In fact patients are asked to eat and drink while they are in the clinic as this aids the process. They are able to chat, listen to music, and move around if necessary as there are hooks for the bag provided at convenient sites in the clinic.

Although EDTA is not a drug and its presence is not toxic to the body, it is nonetheless excreted through the urinary system within 24 hours, bearing with it the chelated minerals, mainly calcium and heavy metals which are the chief aggressors contributing to arterial disease. The average number of treatments given is 20-40, depending on the severity of the arterial symptoms and on how quickly a response is achieved.

At no time are patients incapacitated by the treatment – they are able to carry on their lives as before, and after the first five treatments are usually very much improved, mentally and physically.

A full description of treatment procedures, considerations and effects is given in Chapters 4 and 5. But it is important to note in this introductory passage that chelation does not have to be performed intravenously using EDTA if arterial degeneration is caught in time. Oral (protective) chelation using natural foods and vitamin and mineral supplements is discussed in Chapter 6. There are so many advantages to be gained by starting early.

History of EDTA

EDTA was never formed to chelate metals from the body, but incredibly to chelate calcium stains from textiles which tended to appear due to a reaction between the dyes which were used and hard water. The process was developed in the early 1930s in Germany by industrialists, who because of war clouds gathering, were seeking to develop their own chelating agents rather than rely on imports such as citric acid, supplies of which might dry up during a lengthy campaign.

EDTA was patented in 1935 and was so successful that it virtually replaced the previously-used substance, citric acid. Interest in the substance spread to the United States, and work proceeded both in Germany and in the USA which led to the further refinement of the substance and its eventual adaptation for use as a chelating agent by the food industry, in particular as a stabilizer for canned and bottled foods. (A famous mayonnaise contains it to this day).

EDTA and Lead

It was research originating in Europe in the 1940s (when the possibilities of poison gas warfare triggered a mammoth search for poison antidotes) which led to EDTA's current biological applications. At that time lead poisoning was quite common in certain industries and it was discovered that EDTA could chelate lead from those who had suffered lethal doses of it. (The potential value of this treatment today in respect of those who live close to motorways and have been contaminated by the lead in gasoline fumes is inestimable.)

After World War II, interest in EDTA crossed the Atlantic and resulted in the first real research being carried out at Georgetown University. The result was that EDTA became established in the US as a regular chelator of lead and other poisonous metals, and eventually this led to some interesting clinical observations.

Among the groups of people who were most frequently treated for lead poisoning were workers in battery factories and sailors in the US Navy who painted ships with lead-based paint. Because of their intensive association with a dangerous polluting agent and free radical producer, many also suffered from arterial disease. But once they had been successfully chelated of the lead, it was noticed that many of their arterially-based problems improved dramatically as well.

This led to some lateral thinking which eventually established its value as a reverser of arterio-, or atherosclerosis.

EDTA and Calcium

Since EDTA was seen to chelate calcium just as successfully as it did lead, it became recognized as a treatment not only for lead poisoning but for acute hypercalcaemia, a fact which the FDA (Food and Drug Administration) in the USA recognizes to this day.

In his book *Chelation Can Cure**, Dr E. W. McDonagh, one of the pioneers of chelation therapy in America, points out that as recently as 1970 the FDA referred to EDTA as follows: 'The drug is possibly effective in occlusive vascular disorders and the treatment of pathologic conditions to which calcium tissue deposits or hypercalcaemia may contribute other than those listed above.' He

*Platinum Pen Publishers, Inc. USA, 1983.

goes on to comment, 'At that time our Federal Drug Administration recognized and approved the use of EDTA chelation treatment in circulation diseases. Since then the agency has changed its position, not because there is scientific evidence that EDTA is unsafe, but for political reasons alone.'

According to the remarkably consistent experiences of people who work with EDTA chelation therapy on both sides of the Atlantic today, it would seem that in this instance considerations of wealth are dominating considerations of health (*see Chapter 8*) and there is active discrimination against the treatment.

EDTA: An Emerging Pedigree

Imagine you were back in the 1950s and you had such a serious heart problem that you had been given up for dead by your doctors. Then somebody told you about a last-ditch option which might, just might, do some good. What would you have to lose?

Two of the first patients to have EDTA Chelation therapy were both almost completely incapacitated with calcified mitral (heart) valves when they decided to let the then Professor of Chemistry of Wayne State University, Detroit, Dr Albert J. Boyle, and the Professor of Medicine (of the same university), Dr Gordon B. Myers, try this experimental new therapy on them.

Both had 'a very satisfactory return of cardiac function', reports pioneer chelation therapist, Dr Norman Clarke. Clarke was asked to carry on the research of Boyle and Myers at his research unit in Providence Hospital, Detroit, due to the pressure of work on the initial researchers, and he reports his initial attitude towards and experience of EDTA thus:* 'I knew, having been in cardiology quite a number of years (since 1921) that arteriosclerotic cardiovascular disease was a helpless, hopeless situation for the cardiologist. I had to start by trying to find out whether it (EDTA) was safe: what was the best dosage; were there any side effects, and how would we standardize its use as a treatment?

'The first couple of years we treated only hospital patients

* Walker, M. DPM & Gordon, G. MDM. *The Chelation Answer,* New York, Evans and Co Inc, 1982.

where we had them under excellent control. We started with a rather large dosage (10g) and had some side reactions consisting primarily of signs of a (vitamin) B6 deficiency. Some male scrotums lost a complete cast of skin, but it was absolutely painless and with no sensation of discomfort. After finding the proper dosage of course, all those things have never happened again. And even with those large doses we had no unusual or serious side effects. Ultimately we determined, and for a long time gave, 5g and later determined that 3g was the proper dose.

'In the last 28 years of my experience with EDTA chelation I would say conservatively, because after all those years you don't keep accurate records with all you do, but conservatively I have given at least 100,000 to 120,000 infusions of EDTA and seen nobody harmed...I've never seen any serious toxidity whatsoever. I've only seen benefits...'

Dr Clarke went on to say he had seen benefits in many other conditions besides heart conditions including vascular diseases associated with diabetes (these are associated with peripheral vascular disease, often to the point of gangrene, and with cerebrovascular (brain) senility).

Today, the attestations from doctors practising chelation therapy do not appreciably differ from the words of 90-year-old Dr Clarke (who gives himself the therapy).

Anecdotal Evidence v. Double Blind Trial

The anecdote above has been included as an introduction to how EDTA works because it is so typical of the anecdotal evidence which is inadmissible to medical experts. In the past, it has always been easier to prove that EDTA chelation therapy works rather than how it works – however, some 5,000 scientific papers about EDTA have now accumulated, and new scientific techniques have been able to present their evidence in a more acceptable manner to the establishment through meta-analysis (combining their findings after meticulous scrutiny of admissible papers).

The results of the meta-analysis by L. Terry Chappell MD, and

John P. Stahl, PhD*, revealed a highly positive correlation between EDTA chelation therapy and cardiovascular function (sites other than the heart were not considered). (*See Chapter 5 for a fuller description of this.*)

Evidence is just as strong in support of alleviation of all the following conditions:

- coronary artery disease
- cerebral arteriosclerosis
- intermittent claudication
- diabetic gangrene
- impaired vision
- high cholesterol
- high blood pressure
- scleroderma
- calcific bursitis
- tenosynovitis
- prostatic calcinosis
- kidney stones
- cardiac arrythmias
- heavy metal toxidity
- diabetes
- heart valve calcification
- arthritis
- varicose vein pigmentation
- skin ulcers
- skin colour and texture
- thrombosis
- aneurisms
- tinnitus
- depression

and many others. (After reading them you may deduce another reason why EDTA chelation therapy is having such a difficult job of being accepted – the too-good-to-be-true syndrome.)

This formidable array of improvements however, does not seem so strange when it is considered how vital to health the arterial system is. Extending as it does to every organ and part of the body, it must have multifarious effects on health.

Dr Wayne Perry, the endocrinologist and calcium specialist who is the consultant specialist of the London Arterial Disease Clinic, stresses this aspect of arterial/circulatory disease, that is that any approach to it 'must be multifactorial, which is why the clinic in London is trying to deliver a medical service for the circulation and not just trying to chelate patients'. (*See chapters 4 and 5.*)

This of course makes the job of proving the beneficial action of EDTA by double blind trials (which can only examine one factor at a time) all the more difficult. The fact that each researcher goes off

---

**Journal of Advancement of Medicine*, Vol. 6 No. 3, Fall 1993.

on their own tangent has not helped either. As Dr E. W. McDonagh writes in *Chelation Can Cure* (*see page 144*). 'Clinical research on the medical applications of EDTA in atherosclerosis and cardio-vascular diseases, cardiac arrythmias and digitalis intoxication, heavy metal poisoning, sclerotic diseases, calcinosis and hypercal-caemia, arthritis, hypertension and a variety of other diseases [my emphasis] has appeared in reputable medical journals in the US, France, Germany, Czechoslovakia, Russia, etc. since 1950. Extensive medical bibliographies have been compiled from time to time by the US Library of Medicine...'

As doctors who practise chelation affirm, people get better however many arterial conditions they may have, and it has been clinically observed (by researcher Dr Emanuel Cheraskin MD, another of chelation therapy's pioneers) that the average patient he treated had eight diagnosed conditions.

It seems good but is it safe?

Possibly the most important consideration to anyone thinking of embarking on chelation therapy is its safety. In his excellent book, *The Scientific Basis for Chelation Therapy**, Bruce Halstead MD devotes an entire chapter to the safety aspect of EDTA, meticu-lously examining its toxidity in relation to its benefits and in relation to other substances such as aspirin and nicotine.

He concludes, 'When EDTA chelation therapy is properly administered by a well-trained physician and nursing staff, it is one of the safest major therapeutic modalities available in the chronic degenerative disease armentarium. It is also one of the most rewarding therapies for both the patient and medical staff because of the beneficial results produced. It is encouraging to note that in the combined experience of the chelating physicians in the United States after almost 3 decades (NB written in the late 1970s) of using EDTA, involving in excess of 100,000 patients and more than 2 million treatments, the number of significant untoward reactions is probably less than in any other therapeutic modality.'

*Golden Quill Publishers Inc, Colton, Ca., 1979.

EDTA and the Kidneys

When EDTA was first used to chelate those with lead poisoning (who would have died without the treatment) there were sometimes signs of kidney damage as the lethal lead was passed out through the urinary system. This was probably due to the action of lead on the renal tubules, but in any case the dosage of EDTA used then was far greater than is used now. Also kidney function is now monitored religiously in every chelation clinic. As Bruce Halstead points out: 'In dealing with the subject of toxidity it is well to remember that all chemical agents are toxic if used in sufficient quantity...An outstanding example of this situation is oxygen. Without oxygen a person would cease to live. However the very oxygen which supports life can be lethal under certain conditions. The critical factors are dosage and method of administration...' Nevertheless, patients report that their doctors, when consulted about EDTA chelation therapy, frequently throw up the nephrotoxidity factor as a deterrent, despite the fact that the condition was observed in a completely different context and with seriously lead-poisoned subjects. As Dr Wayne Perry succinctly comments: 'GPs are constantly worried because it [EDTA] could be toxic. EDTA is a good deal less toxic than anything they're likely to throw at a patient!' (In Chapter 5 evidence is presented which indicates that EDTA may even benefit the kidneys.)

As a final comment about the safety factor, here is a list of consumer products in which EDTA is regularly found: mayonnaise and salad dressings, baby food, bottled fruit drinks, flavourings, canned foods (over 50 food companies use it), beer, frozen vegetables, animal foods, plant nutrients, soaps, cosmetics, ointments, bath preparations, hair dyes, pharmaceutical products, pulp and paper. And this list could easily be trebled. As Dr Morton Walker comments in *The Chelation Answer* (*see page 144*), 'EDTA is an integral part of our lives, so it had better be safe.'

Seeking the Treatment

For those wanting to find out if chelation therapy is appropriate for your condition, what is the procedure? Obviously you will have had signs, or been diagnosed as suffering from a circulatory disorder, or suspect you may be shaping up for one. You may actually be taking blood pressure pills or other medication for your condition.

Don't change your drug or other treatment routine in anticipation of a quick solution, it takes time and effort to get alternative treatment, and you have to be prepared to go out on a limb.

However, you are entitled to another medical opinion at any time, and one good thing about chelation therapists is that they are all medically qualified, usually highly medically qualified. Moreover they are usually very special, because THEY too have had to go out on a limb.

Providing you are prepared to pay the moderate fee they will ask, you are entitled to a consultation either by asking your GP to refer you (the best route) or, if you meet resistance, by contacting them direct. There is a tremendous amount of trepidation amongst prospective patients about seeking health advice through any other but the accepted channels. As patients (the very word gives the game away) we have been conditioned to feel guilty about what is our right, to seek professional opinions until we are satisfied about the options available and the course to be taken. Directly or indirectly we pay for our health treatment and the buyer has the power to call the shots.

But this does require learning about your condition and taking responsibility for your decisions. If you were going to invest money in shares, you would want to learn all you could about the company you were funding with your investment. You would want to meet its executives and assess them. Health decisions should not differ from wealth decisions.

Ask for literature about chelation therapy. Ask to talk to one or two patients who have had the treatment. Take time to think about it and discuss the implications of having it with your family. Chapter 7 discusses the very curious situation we are in now in the UK where technically the health minister has said that chelation is available on the national health provided your GP will recommend the treatment and provided your local health authority is prepared to fund it. This may mean fighting for what you want and in the end not getting it unless you are prepared to pay for it.

Taking responsibility for your own health is not easy. But in the final analysis, health is your wealth – your major asset in life.

CHAPTER THREE

SURGICAL OPTIONS IN CIRCULATORY DISEASE: A MODERN APPRAISAL

In Chapter 1 there was a preview of the habits that put you at risk of having a major health crisis, such as a heart attack, a stroke, a thrombosis, a pulmonary embolism, an aneurysm, or any variations of these life-threatening conditions.

In this chapter you will find a review of the various treatments you are likely to be offered from the emergency settings into which such events invariably project you – and the drugs you'll get afterwards.

Heart attacks are the most serious and prevalent of the abovementioned arterial events because they affect the body's main life support system, its circulation pump. Something has to be done and done quickly to contain the damage and keep the pump going. (Strokes can be serious too – as can all of these conditions, but there is less likelihood of a crisis decision having to be made regarding interventive surgery – of which more later.)

If you are the victim of a heart attack, any decision made is unlikely to be one in which you are able to partake unless you have thought about it before and communicated your wishes to a close family member. The pain of a heart attack is excruciating (one casehistory subject described it as 'an elephant standing on your chest with one foot resting on your throat') which does not imply ease in communicating.

Usually it is the spouse to whom the emergency cardiac teams will appeal for permission to operate, and there is more than likely to be an element of do or die about the options presented. Yet Dr Morton Walker avows in his authoritative book, *The Chelation Answer*, that you are extremely unlikely to be given the emergency option which may serve you best: an intravenous drip of a free-radical mopper and calcium-chelating agent such as EDTA. This, he says, would reverse the entire destructive process set in motion by the heart attack and save unnecessary vital heart cells from dying (once dead they do not regenerate).

Before examining the options you will be given – and by current medical tradition they will normally involve a form of heart surgery – it is useful to have some idea of what actually happens to the heart during a heart attack, since this process, according to Dr Walker and others, graphically illuminates what is needed to minimize heart damage, maximize heart stability and begin the process of heart recovery.

What Happens in the Heart

Few people realize what a Trojan the heart is. Each day it contracts 100,000 times and pumps 4,300 gallons of blood (figures are from *Chelation Can Cure* and are therefore US gallons). This is the equivalent of 78 55-gallon barrels of blood, which in any measuring mode is a phenomenal performance.

Being a pump, the heart needs to be watertight and as such it cannot rely on the blood it is actually pumping for its oxygen and nutrients. This it receives from the coronary arteries which traverse its surface. These vital but little arteries are end arteries with few interbranching connections, which is a predisposing factor in coronary heart disease (the chief cause of heart attacks), because if one of them gets blocked there is a limited support network.

The heart's pumping action is a result of (1) the innate rhythmic contractability of heart muscle (samples of which will continue to contract rhythmically in a laboratory), and (2) its internal pacemaker which controls the rhythm of its beats. Two other factors which are essential for maintaining healthy heart function are an adequate supply of blood to pump, and an adequate supply of oxygen and nutrients to support its muscular activities. The correct functioning of the valves which let blood in and out of its pumping chambers is also important.

If any one of these factors fail to meet the physical demands made upon them (usually but not always due to arterial disease) the heart may begin to show signs of strain, though this may not happen until the disease is far advanced (which is why so many first heart attacks are fatal – about two out of five).

Pain (angina) normally felt in the chest, arms and throat is often the first signal that the heart is in difficulty and it is at this point that the sufferer ends up either with a full-scale heart attack, if the condition is severe enough, or with a painful warning that all is not well.

What happens next is critical, because it can either set the sufferer on the road to recovery, or begin a process of spiralling debilitation due to (1) life-draining, purse-draining surgery, and (2) suppressive drug therapy which does not cure the condition but does control the symptoms, making the sufferer believe they are better when they are not. (NB: drugs, such as those which control high blood pressure, may be vital to manage symptoms while one is getting to grips with their cause, but they are not a cure. The condition will worsen unless dramatic diet and lifestyle changes are made – see Chapters 6 and 7.)

The Heart Under Attack

When the heart has a heart attack, what actually happens is the heart muscle goes into a kind of spasm, very like the cramp we all experience when we work our leg muscles too hard. This is due to an inadequate blood supply suddenly becoming a critically inadequate supply.

It is also sometimes due to a build-up of unwanted substances in the heart muscle (fats, toxins, calcium deposits, etc) which quite literally cramp its style, impeding either its arterial-supply system or its electrical pace-making system, or both.

It must be understood that the heart cells are energy-producing factories, as are all body cells. Under the presence of enzymes (organic catalysts) they are able to 'burn' food in the presence of oxygen to produce the energy for life. This main process is called oxidative phosphorylation.

When the heart muscle cells becomes critically starved of supplies and/or increasingly poisoned by metal ion imbalances or clogged by blood which is too 'sticky', altered cell chemistry occurs and this, according to experts such as Dr Morton Walker in his book, *The Chelation Answer*, results in the PH of the cells changing from neutral to acid. This attracts even more calcium ions which, in a vicious circle, block oxidative phosphorylization even further. Also, the presence of excess calcium in heart cells is in itself known to precipitate spasms in the coronary arteries supplying the heart.

So the heart is at the point where, whatever the specific cause of the attack, it needs to be stabilized electrically and chemically rather than attacked further and scarred by invasive surgery.

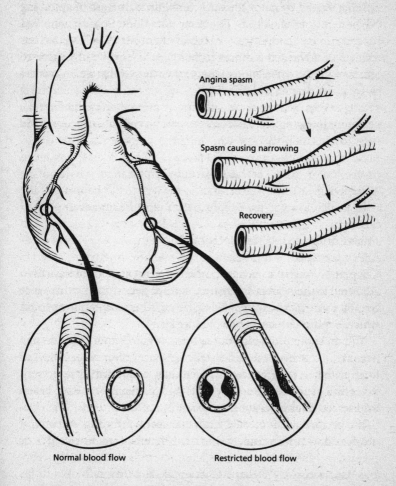

Angina spasm

Spasm causing narrowing

Recovery

Normal blood flow   Restricted blood flow

This, says Dr Walker and others, will arrest the process of starved muscle dying and minimize tissue loss in that most vital of organs. And indeed research has categorically shown for more than a decade* that those who avoid the surgical option when they have a heart attack fare just as well, live just as long (often more actively and usefully because they have not been incapacitated and weakened by surgery) than those who have it.

Only a minority of cases justify heart surgery, and this is an opinion shared by many forward-thinking doctors, such as leading Netherlands cardiologist, Dr Peter Van Der Schaar, who has turned almost entirely to chelation therapy. (Van Der Schaar trained in advanced surgical techniques in Texas but converted almost entirely to chelation therapy when he saw that the results did not justify going on with it.)

That aside, you are more likely to be offered an operation than chelation for some years to come. Although cardiac surgeons could turn to chelation therapy with minimal training (days or weeks, rather than months or years), it takes a lot of persuading to induce a profession to give up at least a part of what for them is a way of life – and living.

Consider how you would fare in the following situation.

Crisis Conditions: What Decisions?

Let's hark back for a moment to the scenario briefly described in Chapter 1. You have had a hypothetical heart attack and have been admitted to the nearest emergency cardiac department (which may be miles out of your way. Worse, it may be an inferior hospital, which is more serious, of which more later).

You, or more probably your spouse, is going to be asked to sign permission for medical staff to take any surgical measures they see fit to stabilize your condition, including major (bypass) surgery. They will especially press for wide permission if you have health insurance. (Never forget that hospitals are commercial organizations: you are not protected from commerce by virtue of being at death's door! British readers who think that they are protected from

*US Veterans study 1977, National Institute of Health Survey, 1988.

this aspect by having a National Health policy are also mistaken: in this instance the commercial interest merely becomes indirect and is based on the size of the desired grant or slice of the budget the hospital can justify by its turnover.)

It is surely wise, therefore, to examine the options which you are likely to be offered, also to keep in mind that you do have one other option – the right of refusal. But this right carries responsibilities and means you will need to know how to discuss alternatives with existing staff who may be pressuring you to give permission 'before it is too late'.

Statistics support your hesitation by revealing that surprisingly few heart attack decisions have to be made in a hurry. They also support you in another way: the risks of dying during surgery or of sustaining serious complications can double (conservatively speaking) depending on the excellence of the surgical team doing the operation and on the standard of intensive care after it, facts which were revealed in a comparatively recent and disturbing survey (in 1988) from America.

Conducted by the Joint Commission on Accreditation of Healthcare Organizations, it found that 50 per cent of US hospitals did not monitor patients properly in coronary and intensive care wards, a percentage which rose still more in the case of regular ward care. Additionally, 35 per cent did not monitor blood transfusions properly.

There were a (conservative) confirmed number of 10,000 deaths from anaesthesia alone, which meant people just didn't wake up from their operations, and nearly one-quarter of all patients left hospital with a condition they didn't have when they entered.

It is difficult to imagine that the situation in Britain would be any better, with the totally demoralizing contemporary picture of closures and shake-ups of key hospitals and disbanding of long-established surgical teams, etc.

Heart Attack Options: The Surgical Armoury

A booklet from the British Heart Foundation (which has a hefty income of £24 million a year and therefore a big say in heart-related policies – largely governed by the cardiac surgeons on its advisory board) outlines the three main surgical and medical options used today:

❧ angiogram (an invasive type of diagnostic technique)
❧ angioplasty (various arterial widening techniques)
❧ bypass surgery (in which blood vessels from other parts of the body are used to form grafts around coronary artery blockages)

There are also one or two non- or semi-invasive diagnostic techniques mentioned, such as electrocardiograms and electrocardiography where soundwaves are used either to indicate heart/artery activity or to detect it (well the latter is non-invasive if they don't ask you to swallow the probe, as they sometimes do).

Let's put them to the test, one by one.

Angiogram (Cardiac Catheterization)

In this diagnostic procedure, a thin catheter tube is snaked through an artery in the arm, neck or leg to reach the heart, pass out through the aorta and into the coronary arteries. Then a dye is injected to see what and where blockages may be.

Harold and Arline Brecher, in their authoritative book on every aspect of modern medical (and other) heart care, *Forty Something Forever*, describe this diagnostic facility as more 'guessimate than science', pointing out that in one landmark study, when 30 angiograms were circulated amongst top diagnosticians, agreement was found amongst them in only 60 per cent of instances. Worse: when the pictures were circulated a second time, the experts disagreed with their original opinions 50 per cent of the time.

They also point out that besides side effects from this painful three-hour marathon, such as nausea, coughing, vomiting, or allergic reactions to the dye (including kidney damage) there can also be serious complications if a piece of plaque gets dislodged from a blood vessel and gets carried to the heart or brain. (Which is why they ask you to sign permission for them to give emergency surgery such as bypass surgery before starting the treatment.)

In *Chelation Can Cure*, Dr E. McDonagh describes one patient who ended up in his surgery with slurred speech, weakness in one arm and loss of memory and mental function. He had been given an angiogram and didn't wake up for three months – bits of plaque were loosened by the exploratory mechanism which lodged in his brain. (He was ultimately treated successfully with chelation surgery.) This is by no means unusual.

Coronary Bypass Surgery

The most important aspect of a heart attack recovery procedure, modern medical experts say, is to limit the amount of damage done to the heart muscle, which can never be repaired. Yet right at this critical moment, while the heart is struggling to recover from its trauma, established medical procedure more often than not performs heart surgery, thus creating more scar tissue and putting a highly compromised patient further at risk from what is a major operation.

Year	Number of CABGS	Number of Angioplasties
1983	180,000	30,000
1986	280,000	130,000
1991	350,000	300,000

In the last 25 years, the coronary artery bypass operation (officially known as CABG or CABS) has become one of the most prolific of surgical procedures. In America, something like a quarter of a million bypass operations are executed each year. In Britain the annual figure is moving towards 20 thousand, which is a lot of bypasses for a country that runs on a severely budgeted national health scheme, especially when the cost of each operation is between $30,000 to $45,000 each (figures are for the USA because they are easier to ascertain but Britain corresponds).

The operation involves:

- sawing through the breastbone, and stopping the heart (before which the bloodstream has to be diverted to an artificial pump which takes over the respiration and circulation functions during the operation process)

➤ selecting and cutting out a blood vessel – either a vein from the leg or an artery from the chest
➤ grafting that blood vessel around (i.e. bypassing) the blockage or blockages in the coronary arteries
➤ restarting the heart with an electric shock

As an emergency procedure following the trauma of a heart attack, this is a mighty load to inflict on a body struggling for life in any case, and as such would need to be totally justified as a life-saving enterprise. Yet there have been many studies to show this is not so, including the previously mentioned Veterans Administration Study, which detected no difference in the rate of survival between those who had bypass surgery and those who did not, 'unless the patient suffered from an obstruction of the left main coronary artery'.

A duplicate study in 1978 by the US National Institute of Health confirmed these findings. Then in the 1980s further studies (the most recent being by the US National Heart Lung and Blood Institute) compared bypass surgery with non-surgical medical therapy and found that bypass surgery achieves no better results in preserving life than conventional drug therapy for the majority of people, severe cases as described in the introduction excepted.

Why is this operation still being done for all and sundry more than 15 years later?

A look at the statistics and reports which have been accumulating on both sides of the Atlantic, especially in the last 10 years indicate that conservatively speaking, 50-60 per cent of bypass operations are unnecessary and/or unhelpful to the condition for which they were done in the first place.

When all the statistical analysis shakes down on this comparatively recent operative procedure (about 30 years in America, less in the UK) it will be seen that far more than 60 per cent of all bypasses performed are not only unnecessary but also damaging to the health of those who have them.

Here are some salient reasons why:

➤ an average of 5 per cent of all bypass operations result in death
➤ over 30 per cent of bypass patients' grafted arteries block within

the first five years, while 10-15 per cent fail in the first year. So, the operation has to be repeated

- over 25 per cent of those having their chests split open experience terribly crippling complications. There are the complications of the leg grafts, causing swollen feet and varying degrees of pain and discomfort on walking, occasioning the need to wear a support bandage on the afflicted leg. Then there are the more difficult to pin down symptoms suggesting neurological damage, possibly, some experts say, due to tiny bubbles of oxygen or other tiny impurities getting into the brain during the time the circulation is on the machine, or other tiny impurities. These are estimated at around 20 per cent

If these figures seem too round, the reader is referred to the bibliography where literally dozens of research papers are listed in many books. The problem with getting exact statistics on bypass or any other surgical procedure is that factors like death rates during surgery vary from about 2-10 per cent depending on how good or bad the surgical unit is that performs the operations. But averages cannot lie, the overall figures are irrefutable, leading to the inevitable conclusions that:

- bypass surgery is bad news (after one or two repeat bypasses the patient is abandoned)
- bypass surgery is bad for arteriosclerosis (evidence mounts that on the suture sites of the grafts arteriosclerosis is actually exacerbated. Furthermore, vein grafts were never built to carry blood under pressure and may fail. As one expert said, 'Bypass surgery is a patchwork solution to a degenerative disease that affects the entire arterial system, not just one or two replaceable blood vessels.')

It must be remembered that bypass surgery not only concerns itself with the coronary arteries, but with arteries in other key sites such as the carotid artery leading to the brain and the femoral/polipteal arteries leading to the legs.

Statistics for these indicate much the same as for CABS. For example, the Hobson study reported in the *New England Journal of*

Medicine 1993 found that in two groups of men whose carotid artery was more than 50 per cent occluded, half of which had bypass surgery and half did not, although there was reduced risk from getting strokes in the surgical group, there was no improvement in the death rate between the groups due to four postoperative deaths and three strokes associated from arteriography (diagnostic technique) from the surgical group.

Furthermore, the main cause of death in both groups was not from a brain-associated stroke but from coronary heart disease!

Neither of the two groups taking part in the study had symptoms – which leads to the question: if a basic tenet of orthodox medicine is that it treats symptoms and that no treatment can be justified unless there are symptoms, why are thousands upon thousands of youngish people in their forties and early fifties (symptomless people who have been screened because of professional or insurance requirements) being given bypass surgery, or angioplasty? Could it be that they are ideal subjects to improve the otherwise grim survival statistics?

The Angioplasty Alternative

Probably as a result of growing awareness that bypass surgery does not resolve the problems of atherosclerosis but rather compounds them, a newer, less dramatic procedure began to gain favour about 10 years ago – a procedure whereby a small tube was inserted into an artery, threaded into position near the unwanted arterial blockage and then inflated (balloon angioplasty), or drilled (directional atherectomy or high speed rotational atherectomy), or even lasered (laser angioplasty).

Sometimes an ingenious brace or metal coil is inserted and left in place (stents) to hold an artery open. There are also laser procedures which actually pierce holes in the heart wall (puncturing a PUMP?) in the hope that nutrient-carrying blood will leak out into the heart muscle and sustain it.

In America balloon angioplasty (percutaneous transluminal coronary angioplasty or PTCA for short) has gained enormously in popularity. Currently some 300,000 (some say 400,000) of these treatments are done annually in the USA. This outstrips even

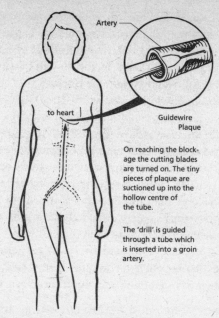

Artery

to heart

Guidewire
Plaque

On reaching the blockage the cutting blades are turned on. The tiny pieces of plaque are suctioned up into the hollow centre of the tube.

The 'drill' is guided through a tube which is inserted into a groin artery.

One of the techniques used in angioplasty

CABS and it is easy to see why. The first is a major operation requiring hospitalization and convalescence of several months. The second requires a relatively brief stay in hospital, virtually no convalescence and can be performed by many more surgeons not qualified to the high degree needed to perform CABS.

To the patient it looks more attractive than bypass surgery, but turning to statistics once more we find that restenosis (re-blocking) of the treated artery re-occurs in 35 per cent of cases *within six months of the treatment*. Considering that much of this treatment is done on young to middle aged patients with symptoms that might as easily be controlled with medication, it seems a risky procedure, especially when there is a 1-4 per cent chance (again the scope depends on how well it's done) of fatality during the treatment, due to guide wires jamming or slicing a flap inside the artery or inflated balloons dislodging plaque.

Some other forms of angioplasty include:

❥ *Directional Atherectomy* (DA) in which plaque is scraped away by a high speed rotational drill. Re-blockage is less than half as frequent as in balloon angioplasty (unless the former technique has been used before it). In 1990, 200,000 treatments were performed in the US and 100,000 in Europe

❥ *High Speed Rotational Atherectomy* (HRSA) which pulverizes plaque

❥ *Transluminal Extraction Atherectomy* (TEA) during which plaque is cut free and sucked out. These procedures are comparatively recent (they were first performed in the late seventies) and so results are in short supply, however they appear to be performing better than balloon angioplasty with less mortality, though laser angioplasty has thrown up some rather sinister early results. Harold and Arline Brecher uncovered a study of 2,000 patients in which 40 suffered a perforated artery, 160 experienced abrupt closing necessitating other techniques being used, 60 required emergency bypass operations, and 40 suffered heart attacks.

With Stents the research does not seem to be encouraging either, due to the fact that they induce bleeding at their site. Since blood thinners have to be taken in order to stop blood from clotting around them in any case this effect must be seen as hazardous.

To sum it all up, the Rand Corporation Study revealed that the procedures of CABS or CBPS, angiography and carotid endarectomy are all significantly overused. Sixty-five per cent of carotid-endarectomies were done for inappropriate reasons, 17 per cent of angiograms, and nearly 50 per cent of bypass procedures.

It may seem inappropriate to inject a note of something as common as sense here, but if one known cause of atherosis is damage to the artery walls, how can it be justified to drill, scrape or stretch them? The scarring alone would surely encourage repair cell growth.

Indeed, a simple comparison of death rates reveals that it is far safer not to have these treatments than to have them. For example, if the known death rate of the average heart patient treated without any procedure is about 1 in 100 per year, a dangerous procedure will only increase that death rate. Based on US figures of 400,000 angioplasty/atherectomy procedures a year here are the comparisons:

- no procedure: annual death rate 1 per cent: total deaths 4,000
- angioplasty: six-month death rate, 4.6 per cent: total deaths 18,000
- atherectomy: six-month death rate, 8.6 per cent: total deaths 34,000

Two other points about surgical techniques such as those described above should possibly be made:

- there has never been a double blind trial to examine their efficacy
- how can a treatment be justified if the reason for it monotonously recurs, eventually rendering the eligibility for further treatment invalid?
- it seems appropriate to comment here that the main reason given by the medical profession for not accepting chelation therapy, despite thousands of positive empirical studies, is...because there have been no double blind trials done.

Drugs in the Treatment of Circulatory Disease

There are an estimated two million people in Britain with high blood pressure. A corresponding figure from America suggests that 40 million people have symptoms associated with arterial disease. Initially most of these will be treated with drugs.

There is no doubt that drugs have an important and useful role to play in the control and management of arterial disease and its many symptomatic manifestations, but to suggest that in any way they are curing the condition is inaccurate.

High Blood Pressure (Hypertension)

There are many purposes for which drugs are taken but this condition is by far the most common. Depending on what doctors believe is the underlying cause of the high blood pressure they may prescribe any of the following categories of drugs:

- diuretics (drugs that increase the flow of urine and thus control the blood pressure by reducing fluid levels in the body

❥ beta blockers (drugs that decrease the activity of the heart)
❥ ACE inhibitors (drugs that act on the kidneys directly)

Studies have shown that there are many side effects to all of these, some serious. For example, diuretics have been shown to elevate blood fat levels of the most dangerous fat categories, thus actually increasing the risk of arteriosclerosis. They also deplete the body of vital mineral potassium and therefore can actually be a precipitating factor in causing heart arrythmias since adequate potassium in the blood is necessary for controlling this aspect.

Diuretics can elevate uric acid levels too, predisposing to gout. They do reduce the effects of too much salt in the system, but a far safer and better way of doing this is to cut out salt.

Beta blockers can have many unpleasant side effects from impotence to affecting breathing function. They also appear to increase the mortality rate when compared to those with the same condition who are not taking them. However they have been shown to reduce the severity of second and third heart attacks and they do control another common symptom of arteriosclerosis – angina.

ACE inhibitors are another part of the large drug armoury for controlling hypertension (high blood pressure) and of them it should perhaps be pointed out that anything that has a direct effect on the body's key organs of elimination, the kidneys, is bound to have effects other than those desired.

In fact this is true of nearly every drug used in this broad area: the advantages must be balanced with the disadvantages, and decisions made based on individual experiences.

Aside from hypertension, the most common conditions which drugs seek to control are: heart pain (angina), palpitations (arrythmia), impaired circulation, sticky or viscous blood, high blood fat/cholesterol levels, and various drugs prescribed for emergency conditions.

The main categories of such drugs are: nitrates (for sudden and severe chest pain), beta blockers (for hypertension and angina), calcium channel blockers (for hypertension or angina), vasoldilators (to improve circulation in the extremities or in the brain), anticoagulants (for those whose blood tends to clot too easily), and antiarrhythmics (for those with palpitations or the reverse, a too-slow heart beat).

Each of these drugs has several trade names depending on what drug company manufactures them and each has a slightly different composition. It is very important that those who have to take drugs know in which category their drug falls, so that if it doesn't suit, others in the same category can be tried.

Just as in any other branch of commerce, some products are better than others. As with commerce, price is very often a guide to quality and those who are prescribed drugs on the National Health may well suffer from restrictions imposed by the constraints of its drug budget.

What usually happens is that doctors are instructed to prescribe the most economical (or locally produced) drug to begin with and if that doesn't suit, than and only then to prescribe one which is possibly superior and more expensive. Not all drugs are available on the National Health and is wise to get acquainted with what is available in your category, because if you are going to take something for the rest of your life (or a considerable time), you might as well try to take the safest most effective product and your doctor will co-operate in this if at all possible.

There is a very good American Publication called *Worst Pills, Best Pills**. There is also a publication in the UK called *What Doctors Don't Tell You* and a small guide[†] to the side effects of drugs.

Drugs in Balance

Chelating physicians also use drugs and may prescribe drugs for patients undergoing alternative therapies for the treatment of circulation therapy in the recognition that (a) people cannot immediately come off drugs and (b) a small percentage may need their support permanently.

What usually happens is that the patient works with the doctor to reduce their drug intake (*see case histories, Chapter 8*). As other measures take effect, the need for drugs goes down. This is espe-

---

*Public Citizen Health Research Group 1988. It can be ordered from Pills, 2000 P Street, N.W. Suite 700, Washington DC 20036.
[†]Available from 4 Wallace Rd, London N1 2PG.

cially true of the need for insulin in diabetes-related circulatory disorders.

Orthodoxy, Heart Disease and Prevention: An Overview

To be fair, it is becoming clear to many practitioners within both the surgical and medical branches of cardiology in the orthodox medical profession that the current modes of treatment for heart/arterial disease do not address the problem early enough or adequately.

Very little prevention has been attempted and this is where major future effort must be directed. Awareness of diet and lifestyle as key factors in the escalation of heart conditions is now becoming more widely accepted, as is the need to address these problems when treating those who have the diseases, not just giving them drugs or surgery.

Heart Attack: Emergency Measures within Orthodoxy

For those faced with emergency heart surgery, are there orthodox treatments which might avoid the risks of invasive treatment modes?

Experts conform that it is not the heart attack which causes heart muscles to die but the starvation of the tissues which ensues in the vital hours and days after it. Harking back to the earlier description of what happens to that part of the heart muscle which has been cut off from its supply of nutrients and oxygen, usually by a spasm or blockage in one of the coronary arteries, it can be seen that distorted chemical reactions occur which attract calcium into the cells which further distorts reactions.

Recent research from the University of Arkansas (and elsewhere) supports the views that many would use an emergency infusion of EDTA at this time, since it is an expert calcium blocker. However there are calcium blockers within traditional medicine which will work too. Dr Morton Walker writes: 'Any one of the chelating agents, such as ascorbic acid, Ringer's lactate (containing lactic acid) or other weak organic acids acceptable for intravenous infusion, will help reverse the process of heart-muscle disintegration and protect the cells against dying, clots from forming, and arrythmias from developing.' He adds, 'of course, EDTA works most swiftly and effectively, however a cardiologist unfamiliar with its application can employ another safe chelating agent.'*

As long ago as 1981 there were orthodox doctors who supported this view. In an address to the Chicago Heart Association in February of that year, Dr Maseri, then Professor of Cardiology at the University of London's Royal Postgraduate Medical School, opined that three-quarters of all bypass operations, emergency or otherwise, were unnecessary. He believed that most heart attack patients could be stabilized just as well with drugs such as calcium channel blockers.

'It is true that arteries narrowed by fatty deposits cause some heart attacks,' Dr Maseri said, 'but there is also evidence of another cause – spasms of the arteries. These spasms, or convulsive contractions, can occur in either narrowed arteries or in arteries free of fatty deposits, and they can be treated by the [then] new drugs.'

Dr Fritz Schellander, who runs the Liongate Chelation Clinic in Tunbridge Wells, in Britain, offered the illustrations presented here as a visual example of this calcium-induced spasm of a coronary artery. His belief, as it is with all chelation therapists, is that ultimately EDTA could be used more in an emergency capacity to stabilize the metabolic condition underlying the spasm. Its prime role is as a calcium blocker but it also has the facility to remove other metals such as iron and copper which sometimes appear as an additional factor during faulty cell metabolism.

EDTA is also safe. When it is considered that EDTA is the solution into which a heart is put when it is taken from a donor, to be kept there until it is transplanted into a recipient, it can hardly be called otherwise.

*The Chelation Way (see page 38)

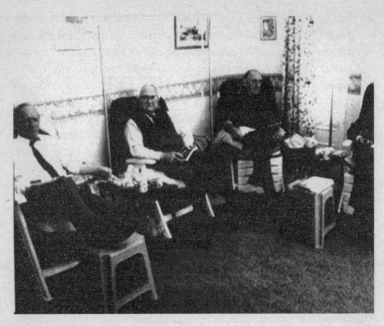

Patients being chelated in the London clinic.

CHAPTER FOUR

TREATMENT MODES: CHELATION, OXYGEN ET AL

The Patient, the Commitment and the Treatment

When a person comes for alternative treatment, they are usually afraid. This is partly instigated by what has been gone through already in the way of treatment, which is often bypass surgery, angioplasty or powerful drug therapy: partly by the gravity of the symptoms (most leave it until very late to try the main alternative, chelation therapy) and partly due to apprehension. There is a great deal of superstition associated with alternative therapy.

Dr Wayne Perry explains: 'It is a big step – a total commitment – which involves considerations which extend far beyond those which are physical to include those which are emotional, psychological and financial.

'In breaking away from traditional medicine the patient may well feel unsupported and alone. As doctors we must never forget that our first duty is to support and comfort the patient.

'Once a patient actually enters the therapeutic atmosphere most are happy to be part of a programme doing something constructive about their condition, and they become part of a treatment environment which lends itself to providing support from fellow patients, also to an interchange of experiences and comparison of progress.'

Most people who seek chelation therapy are well into middle or old age. Although the treatment has great preventative value, symptom-free people seldom come in at this stage unless they have a family history of heart disease. (Hopefully this pattern will change.)

Despite this, and despite the fact that many are high risk patients, British clinics have not experienced a single death during the course of a treatment, which can take six months to a year to complete.

The Protocol of Chelating Physicians

When the patient first makes contact he or she is invited for a series of tests, after being sent a full information pack (with prices) to study beforehand. If the patient has private insurance the cost of tests is usually refundable, but the whole question of cost varies from country to country and is currently a political issue (*see Chapter 7*).

Before beginning treatment, there are several tests required, none of which are invasive or endangering.

- a blood test (for kidney and liver function, as well as a full chemical profile including cholesterol, lipid and sugar levels, and free radical biomarkers)
- an electrocardiogram (ECG or EKG) to test resting heart function
- a urine analysis (a second check for kidney function and for the presence of sugar in the urine (which may indicate diabetes). This is repeated as the course goes on
- a Doppler ultrasound artery scan: to ascertain bloodflow efficiency at 14 arterial sites throughout the body, also to check pulsatility index and stenosis. (NB: Unlike angiography this test is non-invasive and quite painless. After it a print out of the main arterial readings is made on a body map for comparison later
- an exercise stress test to see how the heart performs under exertion (sometimes known as the treadmill test). This test is favoured above the Doppler by many chelating physicians (including Professor Van Der Schaar) because it measures the heart's performance and if this improves then it is clear that the coronary arteries serving it are improving, as will be the entire arterial system

When these results have been ascertained the patient has a full consultation with the doctor who may decide to undertake further tests, depending on the patient's medical history. Blood pressure is taken at this point (and constantly throughout each treatment) and

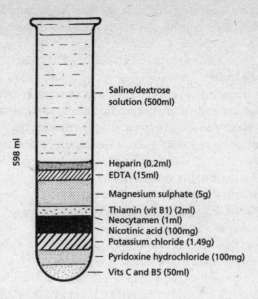

598 ml

- Saline/dextrose solution (500ml)
- Heparin (0.2ml)
- EDTA (15ml)
- Magnesium sulphate (5g)
- Thiamin (vit B1) (2ml)
- Neocytamen (1ml)
- Nicotinic acid (100mg)
- Potassium chloride (1.49g)
- Pyridoxine hydrochloride (100mg)
- Vits C and B5 (50ml)

The contents of a typical EDTA infusion

then a course of EDTA Chelation is recommended, based on each individual patient's need.

The initial course will probably consist of an average 20-30 intravenous infusions of magnesium EDTA. Depending on the patient's tests, the ingredients of the infusion may also include heparin, an anti-coagulant, and various vitamins and minerals known to combat free radical activity, such as magnesium sulphate, thiamin, neocytamen, nicotinic acid, potassium chloride, pyridoxine hydrochloride, ascorbic acid and calcium pentathonate. During the course of infusions the patient will also be required to take an oral chelating supplement both to complement the work of the infusions and to replace any minerals which may haven been chelated out with the calcium (see next chapter for details of oral chelation).

Kidney function is very carefully checked during the course of the treatment, because ultimately the waste products from arterial plaque will be excreted mainly (95 per cent) through the kidneys.

Liver function is also important as the liver helps with detoxification. (Such checks will be constantly monitored throughout the treatment.)

Treatment Mode

Treatment is carried out on an outpatients basis while the patient is fully dressed and comfortably seated in an easy chair. A fine needle is inserted into a vein, usually in the crook of the arm but sometimes in the hand or other suitable site. The drip of 3g (on average) of EDTA, plus other substances as mentioned above, is attached and will take three to four hours to infuse into the body.

This slow entry into the body is designed to achieve the optimum effect from the infusion with the minimum load on the body's excretory organs.

Because of its effect on blood sugar levels, patients are advised to eat something as soon as the infusion begins such as a wholewheat sandwich or some fruit, and frequent drinks are provided to keep up fluid levels for excretory purposes. Directors of chelation clinics are well aware of the care which must be taken when giving fluid to people with some forms of hypertension and allowances are always made for this and other personal aspects which may vary from patient to patient.

EDTA has an immediate effect of lowering blood pressure, and as a great proportion of those who come for treatment suffer from high blood pressure (itself a symptom of arterial disease) then immediate relief from this is sometimes felt.

Towards the end of each treatment Vitamin C is added to the solution in the bag as this facilitates the excretion of the unwanted minerals from the arteries as well as acting as a free-radical mopper and a gentle diuretic.

All signs of the chelating substances have disappeared from the body within 24 hours of the treatment; even so, it is not considered good practice to overload excretory organs as they are ridding the body of toxins which have built up over years, hence it is unusual to give more than three treatments per week and two is more normal.

After the first five treatments patients usually begin to notice early benefits which are experienced by the majority of them, including clearer perception and vision – some patients describe it as 'the head clearing'; an abatement of symptoms associated with high blood pressure (feelings of fullness, tension, ringing in the ears, etc) and a general feeling of more energy and alertness.

However, the main benefits (listed below) are not experienced fully until well after the treatment course is over. Continued improvement is very often noted by patients for at least six months after cessation of infusions, of which more in Chapter 6.

This raises the question of how often chelation therapy should be repeated, for it is not always a simple question of having one course of treatment and forgetting about it (although this does provide long-term remission of symptoms), but rather of maintenance, keeping in mind that most people who come in for chelation therapy do so at a very advanced stage of arterial degeneration.

What many people do not realize is that there is never a time when we can be free of arterial disease in our lives – or as Dr Perry puts it: 'There is no cure for arterial disease.' The process of arterial hardening, by whatever name it is called – arteriosclerosis, athero-sclerosis – is an ongoing one which begins in the cradle and ends in the grave.

But Dr Perry asserts it is not so much the arterial hardening that is the problem, but arterial clogging. This is the contemporary affliction which must be addressed – and the sooner, the better.

Blood Tests

Ischaemia – starvation of the blood supply – is the common charac-teristic of all arterial disease. Blood is a vital factor in the good health equation, and it is to the blood that chelating physicians turn first to see what ails a person displaying symptoms of arterial disease. Dr Perry says: 'Just looking at arterial plaque will not tell you by what process it was caused: but looking at the blood and its composition may give valuable insight into what is going wrong.'

Dr E. W. McDonagh confirms in *Chelation Can Cure*, that 'no two patients will have the same blood chemistries or the same amount of vascular occlusion'.

He goes on to say that a full blood profile (known as a collegiate profile) is required and for this a patient must fast for a minimum of

14 hours. Thus it is normally done first thing in the morning.

The test will reveal, among other things, full kidney and liver function, as well as a chemical profile of blood in respect of certain 'risk factors' in arterial disease such as cholesterol levels, lipoprotein a, homocystine, ferritin, fibrinogen, red cell magnesium and serum E.

Patients are encouraged to learn about these blood components and what the levels mean so that any change registered in future blood tests will have significance for them.

Tests	Range
HDL cholesterol	*Men* 0.8-1.9mmol/L *Women* 0.9-2.2mmol/L (The higher the better. Ideal is over 20% of total)
LDL cholesterol	Under 4.9mmol/L (The lower the better)
Total cholesterol	Under 6mmol/L
Ferritin	*Men* 30-250ng/ml *Women* 30-80ng/ml
Fibrinogen	1.5-4.0g/L
Free homocystine	Under 5umol/L (Ideal is 0)
Lipoprotein a	Under 2.0g/L
Red cell magnesium	1.8-2.7mmol/1rbc (Ideal is over 2.7)
Serum E	0.9-1.6mg/100ml (Ideal is over 1.6)

The table above shows the risk factor aspects of blood tests for circulation problems and the safety ranges into which results should fall.

The composition and condition of the blood will also tell about predisposition to certain kinds of atherosis – too-thick blood – which leads to clotting which in turn leads to thrombosis (too-fatty

The capillaries and arteries as age increases:

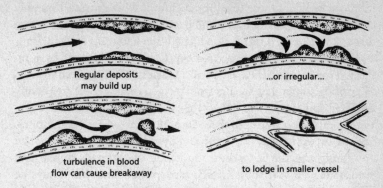

Regular deposits
may build up

...or irregular...

turbulence in blood
flow can cause breakaway

to lodge in smaller vessel

blood leading to clogged arteries). The platelet factor is also an extremely important one (*see Chapter 5*).

The fact that patients often notice a rapid abatement in symptoms is thought to be due to controlling this clotting process.

This rapid improvement is even better understood when it is considered that most patients being treated have turbulent blood flows due to blockages of one kind or another, and according to Poiseuilles's Law of Haemodynamics, in the presence of turbulence in the arterial blood flow it takes something less than a 10 per cent increase in the diameter of arterial walls to effect a *doubling* of blood flow (as stated by Bruce Halstead in *The Scientific Basis of Chelation Therapy*). Thus for this small improvement no less than 50 per cent more blood gets through than before.

Opening the Supply Lines

The importance of monitoring and establishing how well blood is getting through to the tissues is not so much on account of the blood itself but of the raw materials which it brings and takes away. Oxygen must be brought to body cells for fuel to be burned to produce energy for daily life and the results of this combustion (carbon dioxide) must be borne away or they will toxify the system. Regrettably as we age, both the mechanism of absorbing oxygen from the lungs and getting it into the bloodstream diminish considerably, partly as a result of our more sedentary lifestyles (not stimulating deep respiration) and partly because red blood cells become more sticky and adhere together in clumps which means that only those on the outside of the clump become oxygenated on their way through the lungs. The result is a condition known as oxygen drag.

Turning to *The Healing Powers of Chelation Therapy*★ by John Parks Trowbridge MD and Morton Walker, DPM, the authors say, 'The body sometimes suffers from oxygen drag. People frequently don't breathe deeply enough or they live in a polluted atmosphere. For example, cigarette smokers and toll takers at bridges, tunnels and on superhighways suffer from oxygen depletion because they constantly breathe in carbon monoxide in cigarette smoke and automobile exhaust fumes. [NB: carbon monoxide will always be taken up before oxygen.] These people often develop degenerative diseases...'

Quite apart from the fact that twentieth-century lifestyles do not predispose us to breathing in our fair share of oxygen in the first place, our oxygen supply is further compromised by imperfect and inadequate conduction of it to the tissues through narrowed and partially blocked arteries or for the reason above.

One of the actions of EDTA is to restore the function of the transport system of the body – the circulation – thus improving oxygen and other nutrient transport, but this can take time. In the case of severely compromised patients, an additional therapy is being increasingly used to top up depleted oxygen supplies to the cells and give early help to the sufferer. This is known as oxygen or ozone therapy.

Oxygen/Ozone Therapy: Adjunct to Chelation Therapy

The wonders of Hyperbaric Oxygen Therapy were launched in America in February 1990 on the national programme *Good Morning America* by Dr Thomas Buzzoto. In fact the therapy was being practised at the McDonagh Medical Center in Kansas City some years prior to this. In his book, *Chelation Can Cure*, Dr McDonagh writes: 'Hyperbaric oxygen therapy (HBO) is available to the most seriously ill patients, or those who might want to accelerate their

★ New Way of Life Inc., Connecticut, 1985.

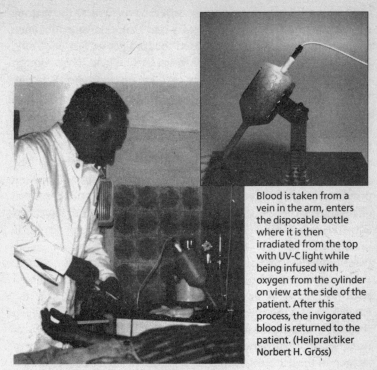

Blood is taken from a vein in the arm, enters the disposable bottle where it is then irradiated from the top with UV-C light while being infused with oxygen from the cylinder on view at the side of the patient. After this process, the invigorated blood is returned to the patient. (Heilpraktiker Norbert H. Gröss)

recovery. The extra boost to the healing process is remarkable. I would compare the difference to that of a jet fighter aircraft when the pilot turns on the afterburner. It really multiplies the speed.'

Sometimes the oxygen is used to 'bathe' a gangrenous limb (caused by the extreme circulation failure associated with advanced diabetes) or an ulcer which does not heal such as on a varicose vein (again circulatory in origin).

Dr Fritz Schellander, who uses an alternative form of oxygen therapy at his clinic in Tunbridge Wells, says that quick as chelation is in giving results, he likes to encourage seriously ill patients in their improvement by immediately administering a course of this therapy.

Dr Schellander, an Austrian by birth, became familiar with oxygen therapies and their useful role in the treatment of degenerative (and indeed infectious) diseases through their diverse use in

Germany, where no less than four different versions of the therapy are commonly deployed by doctors and heilpraktikers (qualified alternative therapists). UK-based heilpraktiker Derek Wolfe, convenor of the first oxygen conference to be held in London in April 1994, uses oxygen therapy in his naturopathic practice in Holsworthy, in Devon. The technique he prefers is one known as HOT, (Haematogenic Oxidation Therapy), whereby a small amount of blood is removed from a vein, suffused with oxygen, and at the same time irradiated with UV-C light for some 15-20 minutes before it is returned to the vein from which it is taken. The simplicity and safety of this form of oxygen therapy has been proved throughout its long use in Germany where the beneficial effects have been shown to be two-fold: arising from the enlivening, anti-free-radical effect of the oxygen and from the catalytic effects of the light radiation. Observations have shown such benefits to persist in patients for some 46 weeks after final treatment.

It must be remembered that oxygen starvation is now thought to be at the base of all degenerative disease in some degree or other, either because the mechanism for absorbing oxygen has flagged (breathing declines with age, stress and insufficient exercise) or because of disturbances and deficiencies in the utilization of oxygen in the cells. Experiments by pioneers such as Professor Dr Manfred von Ardenne have shown that administered oxygen, especially when taken with exercise, can effect a regeneration which reveals itself in blood oxygen levels normally only associated with young people. In particular the heart/lung system is rejuvenated and through it the entire body.

Dr Simi Khanna, who uses oxygen therapy in conjunction with chelation therapy at her clinic in Richmond, near London, believes its effects enhance chelation. She prefers to use ozone in preference to oxygen, though otherwise her method of delivery is essentially the same as Wolfe's. Khanna herself was cured of serious illness by receiving ozone therapy in Germany where it has been practised since 1959. Ozone has known bactericidal, viricidal and fungicidal effects as well as improving blood rheology. However ozone is highly volatile and unstable and must be administered with care.

Its benefits are conferred through this very instability, as Dr Fritz

Schellander explains in an article in the *Journal of Alternative &*
Complementary Medicine, June 1992: 'Ozone is a gas: an energized
form of oxygen with a chemical formula O_3. It is unstable and
dissociates readily back into oxygen (O_2), thus liberating so-called
"singlet oxygen" (O) which is a strong oxidizing agent.' This is the
effect which has been shown to stimulate an activation of the
enzymes involved in free radical scavenging.

'In addition,' writes Schellander, 'ozone can be shown to have a
measurable benefit on the uptake and utilization of oxygen through
improved glycolosis of red blood cells, an improvement in blood
flow...the stimulation and activity of mitochondrial respiration [ie
intercellular respiration] and other metabolic pathways.'

With all these beneficial effects it is little wonder that it is increasingly being used as an adjunct to chelation therapy; the one being
effective in the removal of arterial plaque and the other in
enlivening the newly-cleansed tissues. Together or apart, they
present increasingly attractive alternatives to the more suppressive,
containing-but-not-curing aspects of orthodox therapies such as
the deployment of drugs.

Drug Therapy: Bridging the Gap

Most people are taking drugs when they come in for chelation
therapy. Eventually they may not need them or need so much of
them, but while the healing process is taking place, a series of carefully chosen drugs may be used in conjunction with alternative
therapies.

The following are typical of drugs used by chelating physicians,
mainly in the transitional period:

❥ *Chlofibrate and Niacin.* Used to control high cholesterol levels
 (*but see Chapter 7 for newer, even safer alternatives*)
❥ *Aspirin* in low dose (150-300mg daily). This acts on platelets and
 is probably beneficial in preventing second heart attacks and in
 protecting patients with unstable angina from heart attack. It is
 used after bypass surgery to prevent graft-clotting and in the
 prevention of transient strokes (TIAs). Persantin has a similar
 action and is sometimes used in peripheral arterial disease

❥ *Beta-blockers.* While these do not prevent an initial heart attack, they are thought to be beneficial in preventing a second one. As a result they are usually given after the first heart attack for a period of up to three years. They are also used to control the symptoms of angina (NB: No doubt the factor being controlled here is the worry of having another heart attack rather than an actual improvement in heart function. Beta blockers block thinking brain waves)

❥ *Calcium Blocking Agents* (e.g. Adalat). Since the seventies, these have been widely used for controlling the entry of calcium into cells where it will precipitate arterial hardening, In 1990 Dr Fleckenstein, key researcher into calcium channel blockers, wrote a paper in which he expressed the opinion that up to 40 per cent of the dry weight of plaque can be calcium. But it was never found in the early days of arterial research because the sectioned tissue had already been placed in a decalcifying bath so it could be sectioned more accurately. (NB: Fleckenstein is keen to have chelation therapy researched and has promoted interest in it in the US)

The interactions between drug and chelation therapy and between surgery and chelation therapy are such that EDTA supports but does not prejudice these forms of treatment. However there is ample evidence to reveal that it ultimately replaces them except in an extreme minority of cases.

Surgery

'The protocol for administration of EDTA therapy dictates that we should not accept patients with extreme ventricular failure,' Dr Van Der Schaar elicits. 'Sometimes there is a need to buy time by performing surgery.' US chelating physician, McDonagh expresses the same opinion in different words: 'Occasionally a patient might be seen in an extremely advanced state of coronary occlusive disease and because chelation results might take weeks or months the patient might not have available, surgery is advised. The number of these cases, however, is extremely small.'

Chelation Therapy and Contraindications

It is perhaps timely to discuss this issue here as in certain (very few) instances the therapy is not advised. Van Der Schaar sums it up: 'Sometimes we see it (Chelation therapy) affect renal function and then we tailor the treatment to suit the ability of the patient.' Obviously if renal function is below a certain clearance then EDTA therapy would not be recommended. However, the whole vexed question of chelation therapy damaging renal function – which it does not if the protocol is followed correctly – is discussed in Chapter 5.

Other contraindications are minor personal ones. As Dr Van Der Schaar says: 'Sometimes we get adverse reactions to B3 (nicotinic acid – a vitamin of the B group) when it is added to the drip. Some do not tolerate magnesium in high doses. That's why dose and formula are altered to suit each patient.'

Far-sighted Measures: EDTA and Prevention

Protocol for EDTA chelation therapy is monitored by the American College of Advancement in Medicine (*see Useful Addresses, page 138*) who have declared safety levels for clearance of EDTA in the body. Recently they have modified their protocol to allow the use of mini chelations, using half the amount of EDTA and able therefore to be administered in half the time. This could have benefits in the area of preventive treatment, but not all chelation physicians believe in its efficacy. The latter are of the opinion that it needs a certain concentration of EDTA to effect the removal of calcium from arterial plaque. Time will tell whether this perfectly safe (but not yet proven effective) treatment will have its place. (NB: Another type of EDTA is used from that deployed in regular therapy).

Certainly the role of prevention, and indeed good health maintenance is one increasingly recognized by health authorities all over the world (including the UK National Health System) as being a key issue in future national health programmes.

CHAPTER FIVE

EXAMINING THE EFFECTS

THE 'feeling good' effect of chelation therapy which is described by most people who have the treatment is one of the most difficult to prove scientifically. Double blind trials are concerned with measuring one factor at a time and this is simply not possible in the case of chelation therapy in which a cocktail of chemicals is administered (albeit that EDTA is the predominant one) and in which a spectrum of benefits is registered, including:

- improved mental alertness
- lowering of high blood pressure and its symptoms
- extremities (hands, feet, etc.) becoming warmer
- decrease in anginal pain
- more energy – particularly the ability to walk further without cramps
- improvement in eyesight, hearing and taste
- improvement in spirits
- less breathlessness
- improvement in skin conditions, ulcers, varicose veins
- improvement in sex life

Trying to get to the bottom of what is happening seems to matter a great deal less when you are well again than when you are ill, and following up patients treated with chelation therapy has always been difficult, partly because they get better and go away and get on with their lives and partly because they have come for treatment as individuals, are not part of any health or medical system and have no obligation to cooperate with research. That said, many of them do so out of sheer gratitude for those who have helped them feel better and it is to a meta (compilation) analysis of these patients that we can turn to discover that out of nearly 23,000 cases that were treated for one aspect or another of circulation difficulties (most of them severe), 77 per cent had positive results.*

'Forget trials, chelation is people-proven,' write Arline and Harold Brecher in *Forty Something Forever*. Nonetheless it helps to understand something of what is going on, if only to set the minds at rest of those who may be contemplating a step which is daring in that it flies in the face of organized health care – although even that is inexorably changing (*see Chapter 8*). First let's look at what is being said against it.

Critics of Chelation and What They Say

Your doctor may have heard any one of the following things about chelation therapy:

➤ it doesn't work
➤ it does work but it damages the kidneys
➤ it chelates heavy metals from where they are stored in the body which then circulate through the body and cause damage
➤ besides removing unwanted metals from the body it also removes the minerals which protect the immune system
➤ in the period while it is removing the unwanted minerals it could deplete the immune system for long enough for cancer to occur

Let us take these criticisms seriously. Firstly, the flat statement that it doesn't work.

It is a sad truth that the more general a criticism is, the harder it is to budge from the minds of those who perpetrate it. It is an equally sad truth that we have reached a point in organized health care where the opinions of the patient are not considered to be of value in proving or disproving whether a treatment works for them or not.

Levies of 'empirical, subjective, anecdotary...the placebo effect', are presented as if they render personal experience scientifically or morally wrong. The fact is that chelation therapy does work for the majority of people who have had it, as the meta analysis mentioned

---

*Hancke, C., M.D. & Flytlie, K., M.D. *Journal of Advancement in Medicine*, Vol 6 No 3, Fall 1993.

above has shown once and for all.

In preparing data for the meta analysis the researchers examined no less than 40 published reports about various effects of EDTA on circulation. Only 18 of them met their rigid scientific criteria and yet this still produced the result quoted above.

The researchers went on to say in their report that of the 40 studies examined, only one multi-patient study conducted by Danish *surgeons* showed negative results. (Re-examination of this data has now indicated that their study was flawed – they used ineffective disodium EDTA instead of effective magnesium EDTA. Yet despite this, the British Heart Foundation still cites this one study as sufficient reason not to consider EDTA chelation therapy).

Quite apart from this extremely positive indication that chelation does work on circulatory problems, the general criticism that 'it doesn't work' is completely inaccurate.

It has long been recognized by orthodox medicine that EDTA does work. It is a chelator of heavy metals, including lead, copper, mercury, cadmium, iron, calcium, etc, from the body, and is the standard medical treatment for those with excesses of these metals in their bodies. Organizations as august as the American FDA have accepted its safety for that purpose (proved in the AIMP trial).

Since the technique used to chelate the metals is exactly the same as that which is used for circulation therapy, what is the hue and cry about? In fact EDTA's benefits to the circulation were first recognized as a result and by-product of its being used to treat patients with lead poisoning.

Let us examine the next criticism, that EDTA chelation therapy causes kidney damage. This is more specific and therefore more easily countered.

The allegations are derived from early experiences with chelating those with serious lead poisoning in which very heavy doses of EDTA were used very quickly – it had to be because the threat to life was considerable. As much as 10-20g of EDTA were used in those early chelations, which were often given daily for 14 days. Now the protocol allows for a maximum of 3g per infusion to be given slowly (over a 3-4-hour period) and that a minimum of 24 hours should elapse between each chelation.

Kidney function is rigorously monitored before and during the chelation course and if shown to be at all deficient, a scaled-down amount of the EDTA is used.

In fact there are studies which indicate that chelation therapy actually improves kidney function*. This may centre around the fact that unwanted calcium deposits collect in the kidneys (kidney stones) as elsewhere in the body, and EDTA may act to disperse these. Or it may be because kidney function itself depends on ideal levels of blood pressure operating and if this is compromised by the high blood pressure so often seen in arterial disease then kidney function is also compromised. So, redress arterial disease and you stand to improve kidney function, not compromise it.

The criticism that heavy metals circulate through the body during the 24 hours that it takes for them to be chelated out of it is best answered by looking at the alternative: leaving them where they are. At the moment, it is known that heavy metals are deadly poisons and create havoc with cell metabolism, besides prompting free radical activity. Several studies (for example, Zollinger, Zawirska, Medras) link high lead levels with cancer.

The problems of pollution such as that of lead in petrol are comparatively recent, but studies of individuals living close to fairly busy roads have revealed levels of lead, two or three times those recorded in rural areas.

It is not known at what level lead becomes a serious threat to the immune system, since this would vary between individuals, depending on other factors such as general health, lifestyle, diet, stress, etc. But in 1972 (twenty years ago and automobile traffic has multiplied ten times since then), Dr W. Blumer reports that out of a study[†] of 232 adults living 'in the immediate vicinity of an auto-mobile road, 11 per cent had died of cancer during the period of observation, 1959 to 1970. This percentage was nine times higher than that observed in a traffic-free region of the same community.'

The report goes on to say that the symptoms preceding the onset of cancer (headaches, fatigue, stomach and intestinal ailments,

*Sehnert, K. W., Clague, A. F., and Cheraskin, E. *Medical Hypothesis 15* No 11, pp. 301-4 Nov. 1984.
†Scheiz Med Wach Vol. 106, pp. 503-6.

depression) were mostly alleviated in those residents who were treated with EDTA therapy. As the amount of delta-aminoaevulinic acid in their urine (an early indication of lead poisoning) receded, so did their symptoms.

Reconsidering that EDTA and anything it chelates from the body is effectively excreted within the first 24 hours after the treatment, the risk, even if valid, would seem to be extremely slight in terms of benefits – a risk far far lower than crossing a busy road junction – or having bypass surgery (*see Chapter 3*).

The allegation that EDTA, in removing unwanted minerals from the body may also remove wanted minerals, is reasonable. Firstly chelation therapists have always recognized this as a possibility and have safeguarded against it by providing mineral supplements during the chelation course. However evidence is mounting as the years go by that EDTA is selective in its stripping of metals, only stripping metals where they are unbeneficially placed.

Research pertaining to this effect largely centres on calcium, since its interference in cellular activity in artery walls and its presence in arterial plaque have been witnessed for some time. Concern has always centred around the possibility that whilst EDTA leached calcium from arterial walls, it might also leach it from bones or teeth.

In fact several studies have shown the opposite to be the case. It is only the inappropriately-sited ionic calcium which EDTA acts upon, not calcium bound in bones or teeth. In fact, due to the removal of the ionic calcium and subsequent (temporary) drop of blood levels of calcium, the entire calcium metabolic process is stimulated in much the same way as eating is stimulated by hunger.

The specific result is thought to be stimulation of the parathyroids, which produce parahormone which in turn prompts the formation of bone matter. This process has been described by researchers such as Rasmussen and Bordier (1974), and followed up by Cranton and Brecher (1984) who were interested in finding out why those who had chelation continued to improve and add bone for at least three months after the treatment had ended. The production of osteoblasts (bone cells) was shown to be heightened for this duration. (My own bone-scan test results confirm this – a 3 per cent increase in bone after 17 chelation treatments.)

Attention must also be drawn to a recent study (done in 1993) whose findings are not as yet published but will be by the time this book goes to press. Conducted by a leading Netherlands research organization (IVVO-TNO) it examined, among other factors, the excretion of heavy metals brought about during chelation therapy and noted the interesting phenomenon that although zinc, a vital metal for health, was excreted along with unwanted lead, cadmium and iron, levels of zinc in patients undergoing chelation actually rose as the therapy proceeded. Thus a regulatory mechanism seemed to have been stimulated.

Not withstanding increasing evidence, such as this, that in fact EDTA's action regularizes mineral distribution throughout the body, nor compromises it, provided safeguard measures of mineral supplementation are routinely followed. Still the critics make statements such as, 'the minerals do not get back where they should be.' When this opinion was put before Dr Fritz Schellander, he said, 'This can easily be tested: if a blood test is not good enough, take an intracellular blood test...take a red cell magnesium test...'

He went on to say, 'That sort of general criticism without scientific support is typical of our critics, who can't prove their negative view of EDTA but ask *me* to prove my positive view in each and every way.'

And in any case treatment risk, whatever it may be – and evidence points to it being very much less than that of bypass surgery, drugs or angioplasty – must be weighed against the severity of the illness, in many cases life-threatening, for which the treatment is being given. That point seems to have escaped everyone. No treatment is without some risk, however slight.

Chelation: Its Therapeutic Effects

Turning from the criticisms to the benefits which have been scientifically observed (as distinctive from those which are perceived by patients undergoing the therapy) these centre on the following:

❥ improves and regulates calcium metabolism
❥ diminishes free radical activity
❥ regularizes platelet anomalies, thus diminishing danger of clot-

ting, thrombosis, etc.

- improves enzyme activity
- regulates iron metabolism, thus diminishing lipid peroxidation, considered to be one of the most serious forms of free radical activity
- improves uptake of oxygen to the cells
- chelates heavy metals (now considered to be at least as important as its beneficial effects on arteries)
- controls hypertension, sometimes removing the need for drug therapy
- prevents arterial spasms by its calcium-blocking activity (NB: not strictly blocking so much as controlling)
- stimulates hormone activity (for example, parahormone and others)
- reduces the need for insulin in diabetics
- improves bone metabolism
- reduces the risk of contracting cancer
- improves bloodflow to the brain, heart, legs and body organs
- reduces depression

How EDTA Works

The action of EDTA, like the disease it treats, is multifarious. It seems to have a regulatory action on many vital systems of the body, systems which tend to malfunction with increasing age.

Whether this is because it clears body systems of unwanted debris, thus allowing them to get on with their work, or whether its action is one of chemical intervention, is really irrelevant to the atheroma sufferer. However from the scientific point of view, the main benefits seem to fall under several main categories: removal of calcium, regulation of the clotting factor, stimulation of enzyme production, and last but by no means least, removal of poisons and system suppressives such as heavy metals.

The Calcium Factor

Calcium is one of the commonest minerals in the world. From earliest years we in the west are brought up with a large amount of it in our diets. Instead of beginning with the moderately calcified breast milk and being weaned onto a variety of solids, we are brought up on cow's milk, which was designed for an animal with bones many times larger and denser than ours.

Dairy produce has become a western favourite and many 'treat' foods are composed around it – ice cream, cream itself, cream cheese, fromage frais (give a product a trendy name and sell it all over again), milk shakes, yoghurt drinks and yoghurt itself, cheese in its many forms, etc.

There is also abundant calcium in many of the popular foods we eat (*see Chapter 7*), besides it being in drinking water. But for now let's assume that it is one mineral of which we are not in short supply.

Whether due to excesses in the diet or not, something seems to go wrong with the calcium metabolism around middle age. It is a metabolism which is constantly in and out of play in the body, since blood levels of it have to be kept within a critically narrow band, and to achieve this, thyroid and parathyroid hormones work in balanced opposition to each other, secreting hormones (calcitonin and para-hormone) which stimulate the release of calcium from body stores, such as bones, or suppressing this activity by releasing hormones which stimulate calcium to be laid down in bone.

Calcium therefore moves from easily transportable states which dissolve in blood to non-soluble states which can then be stored. It is this transportable ionic calcium which largely becomes part of arterial plaque and incidentally can become part of other calcified deposits in the body such as those around joints and old injuries. It is then known as metastatic calcium. (NB: ions are atoms or groups of atoms which carry an electrical charge, either positive or negative, of which more later.)

The minerals of the body work in harmony with each other but also in juxtaposition – so that one is balanced against another to achieve metabolic results. If the diet constantly provides excesses of one and deficiencies of another, then mineral imbalances occur and the body somehow has to cope with this by finding storage places for the excess and attempting to overcome problems caused by the deficiencies.

This is what is thought to happen when the body starts laying down calcium on artery walls. There is another hypothesis which suggests that this happens because the body 'perceives' that the arterial walls are becoming injured (by the action of destructive free radicals) and hence it deploys calcium as it does in other injury sites, to shore up the damage. Whatever the reason, the result is an accumulation of deposits which block circulation and prevent reabsorption of other plaque components that get shored up as well, such as fats, blood cells (especially platelets which are also used for repair purposes) and fibrous material, such as elastin and collagen.

Ionic calcium is of great importance in the function of the heart and other muscles of the body. The body is an electrical system and heartbeat is produced through the interplay of positive and negative ions within and without body cells which create what is known as an electrical potential across the cell membranes. This stimulates heart (and other) muscles to contract rhythmically because of a constant reversal of the potential.

Bruce Halstead writes in *The Scientific Basis of EDTA Chelation Therapy* that 'there is an increasing amount of evidence that an abnormality in calcium metabolism is the biochemical lesion primarily responsible for heart failure'. He goes on to say that the lesion is believed to be caused by a difficulty arising in the exchange of the action potential involving calcium ions due to problems in the conducting cell membranes.

What this all amounts to in lay terms is that heart attacks can and do occur because of a faulty calcium metabolism on two levels: firstly, on the accumulative level of progressive calcification of arteries, including coronary arteries, and secondly, on the muscle spasm level due to the malfunction of heart cells themselves. Keeping in mind that mental and emotional input also affect this most sensitive organ and you may have the situation of a heart attack occurring (*see Chapter 3*) where there is no significant blockage of the coronary arteries. All the more reason to get to grips with the causes, be they metabolic and therefore probably dietary (*see Chapter 7*) or stress-related (*see Chapter 6*). But there are one or two other factors in this complex equation worth mentioning.

Cells and Cell Membranes Undermined

As stated before, cells produce the energy for life. If we feel tired, it is because we have dipped too deeply into our energy bank by overdoing things or because there is a malfunction in the energy production line. This is dangerous, because a body without energy reserves is a body without defence. A compromised immune system fails to destroy cancer cells, a job it normally does on a regular basis as they arise. A compromised immune system fails to conduct the body repairs needed to maintain integrity of its systems.

One of the ways in which a system can be compromised is by the destruction of its tissues by free radicals. These particularly affect the cell membrane – that is, the semi-permeable protective wall, which needs to perform well in order to let oxygen and nutrients in and carbon dioxide and toxins pass out. Cell walls are largely composed of fats (lipids) and, if these fats become oxidized, they change their quality as surely as culinary oils and fats do when they become rancid.

Heavy metal ions prompt this destructive process – especially iron (another excess in our diet caused by a high-protein intake far beyond a body's needs, especially in later life when exercise/activity levels drop dramatically), but also copper and calcium.

This destruction of cell walls could be likened to a picketed factory where raw materials were not getting in or finished products

Lipid peroxidation (free radical activity). Membrane → organelle damage → cell damage → disease

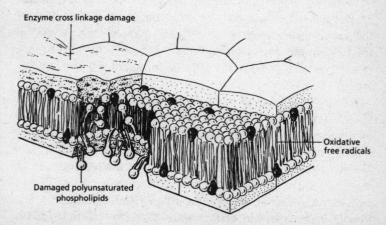

Enzyme cross linkage damage

Oxidative free radicals

Damaged polyunsaturated phospholipids

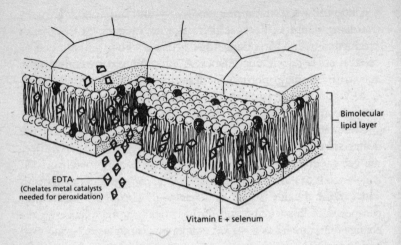

EDTA protective mechanism

out. Inside, at the assembly line, the mitochondria, or tiny energy producing units, attempt to make do with what is there. One of their main functions is to convert inorganic phosphate (ADP), sugar and oxygen into adenosine triphosphate (ATP). This energy-producing activity involves a chain of complex biochemical steps which are themselves dependent on an army of enzymes (organic catalysts) to make this burning process happen at body temperature.

If, for any reason, cell membranes are compromised, then ATP production falters and cells become energy-starved. This makes them more acidic which in turn attracts yet more ionic calcium into the cells. In the case of muscle cells (such as in the heart or in its coronary artery walls) this is a classic formula for them to go into spasm.

Exactly what cocktail of causatory factors actually triggers the spasm differs with each person. It may be free-radical activity damaging cell membrane walls, dietary imbalances or oxygen deficiency caused by a poor blood supply (or poor breathing). A classic cause is thought to be an imbalance between calcium, an inhibitor, and magnesium, an activator, since these two metals must balance each other in order for the cell to maintain its healthy function. (Western diets contain far too much of one – calcium – and far too little of the other – *see Chapter 7*.)

Calcium-channel blockers act to prevent absorption of inhibitory calcium ions into the cells, which is why they are so widely used today, but they do nothing to cure the underlying condition nor do they cure the energy deficit which also underlies it.

EDTA is actually capable of removing inhibitory ionic calcium from the cells, thus allowing the cells to resume energy production. Whilst removing excess calcium, it also removes other heavy metals which may also be interfering with cell activity such as iron, lead, cadmium, mercury, copper or even aluminium.

The Platelet Factor (*see also Chapter 4*)

Another troubling characteristic in the atherosclerosis process is the tendency for platelets to aggregate around injury sites in arterial walls and form clots. This is an expression of a natural healing function of the body, but being taken to an extreme. Furthermore when it is being conducted in arteries, especially tiny arteries, then such sites are likely to become clogged by such activity.

This is made even worse by the tendency of platelets to change their shape from round to pod-like and to develop hair-like filaments – all this to stem bleeding at injury sites in arterial walls.

But, as Bruce Halstead writes, 'although the clotting process is essential for the control of haemorrhages, it can also be life-threatening when it takes place on the walls of distressed coronary or cerebral arteries.' Coronary thrombosis or cerebral thrombosis are the results of such mismanagement of a healing function.

EDTA is known to control this process by occupying sites on the artery walls to which platelets would normally attach themselves. It also regularizes their shapes, making them slip past injury sites rather than adhere to them. This, Dr Van Der Schaar and others consider to be one of the major roles EDTA plays in the control and regression of atherosclerosis. Orthodox medical treatment prescribes blood-thinning drugs for this condition such as warfarin or aspirin, but neither remedy addresses the source of the problem.

The Heavy Metals Factor

Dr Fritz Schellander believes that the action of EDTA on ridding the cells of their heavy metal load is even more important to health than that of removing calcium. He says:

'If you look at illness patterns in society now it can be seen that they are changing. Younger and younger women are getting endometriosis and ovarian cancer. ME and AIDS are rife, leukaemia has increased enormously...whereas GPs used to cope with a patient list of 2,900 patients, now they cannot cope with 2,200 patients.

'Ecological disasters are going on and they are unprecedented and where they are unprecedented we don't know how to deal with them.

'Heavy metals may not have reached toxic levels but they are still there undermining health. Every young mother who gets pregnant now has significant levels of lead – this seeps straight through the placenta into the unborn.

'If you were to introduce one twentieth of the toxic dose of whisky into a newborn and kept doing it you would end up by aged seven with a rather dumb child...

'Then there's cadmium. Cadmium is the by-product of many industrial processes today. It is now in the soil of many industrialized countries.'

We are reminded that mercury is another deadly poison which is in dental amalgum. Until recently mercury ointments and tinctures used to be on sale – now this practice is largely dying out.

Four poisons which Schellander cites that have a particularly bad effect on the body are lead, aluminium (which features in Alzheimer's disease) mercury and cadmium.

He believes that chelation therapy, unaccepted as a remedy for circulation, should be promoted and used in its medically accepted capacity as a chelator of heavy metals. In this respect he says, 'It's not unorthodox, it's not unconventional – and it's not new.'

In an article he wrote for the *British Journal of Alternative & Complementary Medicine* (October 1992) he stated: 'In view of all the evidence for the effectiveness of EDTA as a chelating substance it seems mandatory that its role as an important detoxifying agent be assessed by major research institutions.'

He points out that the heavy metal burden 'which we all unavoidably suffer in an industrialized society' appears to rise with age. By midlife 'levels are even to a sixth or an eighth of an acutely toxic dose.'

It is well known that levels of lead in the blood are linked with increase in cancer mortality – which brings us to another very interesting benefit to be had from EDTA chelation therapy.

The Enzyme Factor

Enzymes play a vital part in maintaining the integrity of the arterial walls. Enzymes are organic catalysts which enable chemical processes to take place at body temperatures. These enzyme activities are quite efficient in youth but, according to Morton Walker and others, 'starting in the fourth decade of life, they begin to diminish in supply to about one-half of their previous activity'.

He goes on to describe how this reduction decreases the repair process of arteries which in turn leads to overcompensatory activities which encourage the aggregation of cholesterol and calcium to form plaque. This in turn attracts platelets which collide with the plaque and in response to the perception of injury, release their own hormones, which in this case are likely to be the ones which prompt coagulation.

Bruce Halstead explains that enzyme activity depends on metal ions for its completion and any distortion in the balance of these is once again likely to promote degenerative activity in the cells. The balance, he says between calcium and magnesium, if distorted (back to dietary imbalances again) leads to excessive calcium concentration which leads in turn to further inhibition of enzymes. This may result in damage to cell function, respiration, and produce an oxygen deficiency state (anoxia) all of which is conducive to chronic degenerative disease.

He also notes the resultant reduction in enzyme activity in artery walls: 'Enzymatic analyses have shown (Kirk 1959, 1968) that of the 98 enzyme systems in the artery wall, 46 of them are in a state of depressed activity in arteriosclerotic tissue.'

He believes that the decrease in arterial enzyme function is part of the picture of aging. He describes how calcium builds up in the arterial lining as a result of an influx of fats which change from fatty acids to insoluble calcium fatty acid complexes, that is, plaque.

He goes on to say, 'These are important biochemical events in atherogenesis and provide important target sites for the action of EDTA therapy in the removal of calcium and other transitional metals, and aiding in the normalization of enzymatic homeostasis.'

This would seem to add weight to the opinion expressed by Fritz Schellander and others that a prime action of EDTA is removing unwanted metals so that regeneration can take place. Schellander goes further and suggests that the excessive presence of calcium in arterial plaque is in fact part of the body's attempt to heal: 'The protective function of calcium laid down around tuberculous lesions or inflamed tendons is well-accepted. Could there be a similar mechanism operating in our arteries?'

EDTA and Cancer

Dr E. W. McDonagh, a respected Kansas City, Missouri physician who has chelated approximately 25,000 patients over the past two and a half decades, decided to run a check on his patients to see how many of them had contracted cancer. (Bear in mind these were people ill with arterial disease when he treated them and in the middle to upper age groups.)

According to the national average, one in three people contract cancer at some stage in their lives. By this average, it was possible that 7,500 of his patients may have contracted cancer. In fact he discovered that only one had done so.

The previously mentioned study* *(see page 71)* by Dr Blumer of Switzerland and Elmer Cranton found a 90 per cent reduction in the incidence of cancer in a group of patients who had received 15 chelation treatments, when compared with a control group 18 years later. All had been exposed to comparatively high lead levels from a busy trunk road. So it could be expected that their incidence of contracting cancer should be higher, not lower, than the national average.

The Diabetic Complication

Diabetes is one of the most rapidly growing afflictions of the modern world. Although the discovery of insulin has stopped people from dying of the illness, the effects of the disease on the circulatory system remain extremely severe. Diabetics have always been in danger of suffering from poor peripheral circulation, which can lead to gangrene, and ultimately to amputation – which is the only final solution recognized by orthodox medicine.

EDTA not only regularizes the actual disease, enabling diabetics who have been treated with infusions to decrease, and sometimes discontinue insulin supplementation altogether, it also restores circulation in the peripheral arteries and prevents the terrible onset of gangrene and its ultimate progress to limb amputation.

Dr E. W. McDonagh writes in *Chelation Can Cure*, that figures from the Nutrition Research Laboratories, Department of Preventive Medicine, Washington University, indicate that the prevalence of diabetes is increasing in the United States at a more rapid rate than the growth of the total population. Although 50 per cent of diabetics have inherited their tendency towards the disease, it doesn't have to be constellated unless circumstances such as diet, lifestyle, allow it to be.

McDonagh notes that over 80 per cent of the US diabetics are overweight. It would appear there is a link between diet, faulty carbohydrate metabolism, lowered amounts of vitamin C and the development of the diabetic syndrome. Whatever the cause (*see Chapter 6*) diabetes is associated with many other chronic degenerative diseases and its increase is linked to western countries and their diet and lifestyle characteristics.

Dr McDonagh has pulled some diabetic patients right back from the brink of death by giving them chelation therapy.

In England, the Liongate Clinic and the Arterial Disease Clinic, have both independently offered to treat with chelation therapy those facing leg amputation because of compromised peripheral circulation, either through the diabetic syndrome or other causes. To date no health authority has shown interest in experimenting with these hopeless cases (*see Chapter 8*).

Summary of Benefits

EDTA removes chromium, iron, mercury, copper, lead, zinc,

cadmium, cobalt and aluminium from the body – in that order. In fact it is interesting that there are less studies which prove its effective removal of calcium than of other heavy metals.

Metals chelated by EDTA (in descending order)	3) mercury 4) copper 5) lead 6) zinc	9) aluminium 10) iron (other forms) 11) manganese 12) calcium
1) chromium 2) iron (some forms)	7) cadmium 8) cobalt	13) magnesium

Two or three recently discovered benefits centre around the removal of iron and copper, two of the most destructive, free radical producers in the body. Apropos of this facility, research has shown it to have a striking effect on hyperactivity in children caused by exposure to lead. It enhances the heart muscle's phosphorous utilization, therefore improving heart function. And it effectively removes cadmium from tobacco smoke which is known to compete with zinc, a vital requirement for enzyme activity.

EDTA could become a valued remedy for controlling the effects on the circulation and other body systems of unprecedented toxic loads characterized by our twentieth century life on a polluted planet.

EDTA and Orthodox Interest

Has EDTA elicited any speculative or investigative interest from within orthodox medicine about its effects on arterial disease, with particular relevance to the crisis confronting medicine to find solutions to disease of the coronary arteries?

In 1993 Meridian (Southern UK) TV made an interesting documentary on chelation therapy and invited professor Richard Vincent, Consultant Cardiologist at the Royal Sussex County Hospital to provide an orthodox comment on the work of chelating physician, Dr Fritz Schellander, of Tunbridge Wells.

Professor Vincent is Professor of Medical Science at Sussex University and his interest in EDTA therefore stems both from medical and scientific sources:

'The proposed logic that chelation therapy works by removing calcium from the walls of the arteries is one which conventional medicine finds difficult to see in terms of logic.

'Calcium deposition is slow, therefore its removal is not likely to be quick. One sees coronary arteries cut at post mortem and the scissors go *crunch*. It's a very solid compact piece of plaque. Removing that would make the artery more pliable but removal would be slow, whereas chelation therapy seems to go quicker.

'However calcium is part of the (atherosclerotic) lesion so just dealing with one aspect may help but it doesn't address them all.

'Calcium seems also to be involved in clotting – and blood clotting is also involved in the way these lesions are developed...EDTA might affect calcium and its utilization in clotting as a separate mechanism. My scientific colleagues don't all agree with this but I'm not sure it's been fully investigated.

'Also not investigated, as far as I know, is the possibility that EDTA has an effect on red blood cells. These, in order to get through smaller blood vessels, actually have to squeeze their shape and in a disease like CHD we know that they become less compliant, don't like squeezing down.

'Maybe there's another mechanism at work by which cells are being made more pliable to go through smaller blood vessels into profusion...

'There could also be an effect like one of those groups of pharmacological agents, such as calcium channel blocking drugs...I don't think we fully know about these mechanisms, there may be something there.

'We don't fully know how that (or other aspects) of EDTA would relate to such a long-term benefit from a short-term treatment. In terms of underlying theoretical premise it becomes difficult to validate.

'We see EDTA as a global set of treatments and that makes it more difficult to discern the single agent.'

Back to complexity, which reductionist science finds the most challenging of all concepts to run through the double-blind trial procedure which can only test one thing at a time.

What is good to know is that in more broad-minded orthodox camps EDTA is receiving attention.

Depression and EDTA Therapy

One of the most health-sapping conditions is depression, made worse by feeling guilty about having it in the first place. Depression is an illness, which depletes the body's immune system as surely as would an attack of 'flu or any other infection.

Unfortunately depression often accompanies ill-health, because ill-health renders a person less able to cope, which sets up a vicious circle of disempowerment, since being depressed about this will deplete stamina and mood further.

EDTA does improve depression, whether by the action of making a person feel better physically or whether by the almost generally-felt benefit of 'clearing the head'. A lifting of the spirits often accompanies an improvement in health, so the effect is probably a spin-off from removing the toxic load from the body and clearing its pathways.

However, the effect is proven by the required scientific protocol of today as one over and above any placebo action.*

This is not to suggest one should have chelation therapy to cure depression, but none would deny that it is a worthwhile, not-so-side benefit.

*Kay, D. S. G., Naylor, G. J., Smith, A. H. W., et al. *Psychological Medicine* Vol. 14, 1984 pp.533-9.

CHAPTER SIX

SUPPORTIVE SELF-HELP MEASURES AND OTHER TREATMENT OPTIONS

MAINTENANCE and management of circulatory health depends largely on each individual's particular needs and problems, once the main thrust of the controlling therapies (such as chelation, ozone, etc.) have played their part.

After stabilization, choices widen considerably, and may include regular courses of supportive therapies such as some of those described below, or the more direct route/exploration of how to achieve reduction of stress, since this has to be considered a major factor both in the control of existing arterial disease and the prevention of its recurrence.

Management of stress will also help with subsidiary measures such as in giving up smoking or drinking to excess or quitting eating a favourite food which is known to be bad for the circulation.

In both orthodox and alternative circles, stress management for those with arterial disease is being recognized as one of two major health issues once the disease has been brought under control. (The other is diet or nutrition to which an entire chapter [7] has been devoted.)

Most people recognize that the reduction of stress is important, but think it arises only as a result of pressures from work, relationships, family or financial pressures, not realizing that in fact the body recognizes stress from no less than four different sources. Examining them all can pin-point an unsuspected source of problem.

❥ Chemical stress (such as air pollution, radon gas, pesticides, cigarette smoking, fumes incurred while travelling to and from regular employment, as well as internal sources such as alcohol

consumption, drug taking – including prescribed ones such as chemotherapy – even anti-stress drugs such as sleeping pills and tranquillizers!)
- Physical trauma. Having an accident, a fall and injury, or a surgical operation, such as bypass surgery
- Infections. Anything from colds and 'flu to ME and AIDS
- Emotional stress (marital problems, employment problems, financial problems, family issues and responsibilities)

The first three categories of stress may be more difficult to avoid since they are occupational and environmental: however, protective measures should be taken wherever possible, such as installing air or water purifiers in the home and taking great care in the choice of household cleaning agents, sprays, and garden products, so that safer forms are favoured to those which are more toxic. (The cardioneurological system is particularly vulnerable to neurotoxic chemicals whether from pesticides, pollutants, such as lead in drinking water, or food additives.)

Noise pollution is a stress factor as well and as much care as possible should be taken to minimize it, and if it affects sleep, try getting used to ear plugs.

Physical trauma is sometimes unavoidable (or seems that way – actually we are far more accident prone when we are tired so we should be more careful then), but much can be done to protect oneself from minor (and major) infections by daily doses of sufficient supplies of protective vitamins, such as Vitamin C, and minerals (*see Chapter 7*).

How Type A (high achievers) achieve Heart Disease

The fourth category of stress is more difficult both to quantify and to control. But it would appear that circulatory diseases and disorders happen more often to a certain type of individual, one who could be classified as a high achiever. People of this kind are commonly referred to as 'Type A's.

John Buckley, Director of the Arterial Disease Clinic in the UK, makes the point that it is this 'Type A' kind of person who, when being treated with chelation therapy, doesn't want to complement the treatment with the lifestyle changes the clinic recommends. This in itself is typical of Type A (don't-mess-with-me-and-my-lifestyle) behaviour.

Type A people seem to predominate in the arterial disease profile – to such an extent that Dr Van Der Schaar, who has been working with circulatory problems for most of his professional life (and only recently with those who have other illnesses such as cancer) was initially amazed by the personality differences between his circulatory disease patients and others.

It was Dr Meyer Freidman who first described these in his book *Type A Behaviour and Your Heart*. This classic is still worth reading as is anything by Dr Dean Ornish, Professor of Cardiology and Internal Medicine at the University of California. The latter has concentrated particularly on achieving the regression of arteriosclerosis symptoms using diet and stress reduction only, and has achieved a large measure of success by those means.

Type A behaviour is characterized by the following:

❥ hurry sickness
❥ score keeping
❥ obsession with numbers (especially number 1)
❥ insecurity
❥ hostility and aggression

Unfortunately all of these traits cause the body to run at a fast pace all the time, without a chance to recover, slow down and take stock. Supplies of the hormones released in response to stress, such as cortisone, quickly become depleted, as do supplies of other stress-reactive hormones, such as those from the thyroid gland.

Body repair work gets sidetracked and the person becomes exhausted, although hyped up. This pattern goes on until the hyped-up person finally runs out of steam and enters the countdown period prior to a total breakdown in health, such as a stroke or heart attack.

Angina is commonly suffered by type A people, as is high blood pressure and the tension headaches often related to this. These become worse until breakdown point is reached (*see the exhaustion curve*).

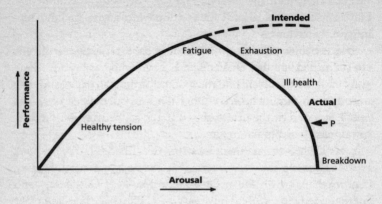

P = The point at which even minimal arousal may precipitate a breakdown

Hyperventilation and Your Heart

British heart specialist, Dr Peter Nixon, has particularly interested himself in the phenomenon of hyperventilation (overbreathing), another classic reaction to stress and one that is extremely bad for the circulation. Thoracic (chest) breathing is known to be associated with stress-induced illnesses and symptoms such as high blood pressure, high cholesterol levels, head symptoms such as dizziness, an inability to concentrate, angina and coronary artery spasms, etc.

The process behind hyperventilation is as follows: breathing through the chest is associated with hurry, tension, rising to the occasion: in other words it stimulates the sympathetic nervous system which responds to our challenges in life.

Breathing through the stomach and from the diaphragm is associated with release from pressure, normality in life, being relaxed and at ease. This is the relaxation response which balances the former response and is activated through the parasympathetic nervous system.

These two branches of the autonomic nervous system should keep us in balance so that we can rise to occasions when needed and react quickly or be at rest and recovering in between. It is called the fight and flight response.

If one side is being activated all the time by rapid breathing, then the body becomes exhausted and unable to rest and recover. Furthermore this habit alters the ratio of oxygen in the blood to carbon dioxide and this actually has some very unpleasant side effects to circulation in the brain.

Arteries are narrowed under this impulse and the blood supply is compromised. Unfortunately, this is one response which may have been learned during youth when so many of us were told to 'put out your chests', and 'pull in your stomachs'. Watching a young baby breathe will provide ample proof of what is natural for the body.

Leaning the Right Way to Breathe

Fortunately correct breathing can be re-learned very simply by lying down somewhere flat and placing your left hand on your chest and your right just below the navel.

Breathe as you do normally and note which hand is rising and falling. After a minute or so, as you exhale press down gently with your right hand and then as you inhale again, allow the air to push the right hand upwards. Keep doing this for a while until you feel the site of the new rhythm.

This is the correct way to breathe and it can become a relaxation exercise if the following steps are added: as you breathe out, count to four slowly: then breathe in, also counting to four. Do not hurry and try to keep the breathing pattern smooth. Note any thoughts which may arise as you establish this pattern and instead of worrying about them, just refocus on your breathing...let the thought go. Don't force it out of your head: just favour the breathing.

Breathing is a very special process in that we can consciously alter it and direct it, or we can completely forget about it and we still breathe automatically. As such it provides a valuable access point to the unconscious part of the brain, where any traumas and emotional experiences may lie which have caused us to respond, like Pavlov's dogs, to certain patterns of arousal. By re-establishing a relaxed breathing pattern we are actually accessing, influencing and controlling patterns of arousal which normally influence and control us. This is the basis of many anti-stress techniques, such as meditation.

Meditation: a Drug-free Way of Controlling Stress

In the 1960s a wave of awareness of other, eastern values swept into the west and brought some of us, quite literally, to our senses.

In the cerebral west we had values which were to do with developing academic gifts: in the East they have always known that all three aspects of the personality must be served, body, mind and spirit, for homeostasis (stable health) to be preserved.

One of the best and most accessible methods of learning meditation comes from the East. Called TM, Transcendental Meditation, it requires the learning of a simple, 20-minute routine of relaxation morning and evening.

There have been so many scientific research papers proving the value of relaxation by this technique to all systems of the body that it hardly bears writing about any more. In 1993, 136 doctors wrote to the UK Health Minister asking that it become available on the British national health scheme, they felt its value as a relaxation technique to be so great.

TM can be learned locally all over the western world, the network is excellent, the training is short and the benefits are long. Look them up in your local telephone directory*.

Versions of such measures as those described above are deployed by clinics specializing in circulation disorders and they usually have their own referrals to experts in their area who conduct this vital part of the protocol. There is no point in getting better if measures are not going to be taken to stabilize the improvement. You cannot walk away from your body, and especially not its psychological aspects which can make all the difference between stability and decline. (NB: If techniques for organized relaxation do not appeal, buy tapes of funny movies or comedy series and watch them each day – laughter IS the best medicine, especially for Type As – and that's been proven in Sweden.)

Giving up Smoking

This should be easier once the above measures have been understood and incorporated into the lifestyle, since stress control is one

*The national enquiry number in the UK is 0800 269303.

main reason for smoking in the first place.

Giving up is not suggested here as a moral issue: the plain facts are that smoking releases millions of free radicals into an already overtaxed system. It also induces the production of something called thromboxane, which makes blood vessel walls sticky. It also makes platelets sticky and is one of the major exacerbators of atherosclerosis and cardiovascular disease.

The action of nicotine on the cardiovascular system is to elevate blood pressure (which is usually on the high side anyway) by 5-10mg of mercury and increase the heart rate by as much as 20-30 beats per minute. In other words smoking pushes the body. That's why it's so hard to give up, together with coffee, because of the artificial feeling of being hyped up and in control.

One of the worst effects of smoking is the effect it has on peripheral circulation. Plethysmographic tracings of digital (finger) arteries show an incredible 400 per cent reduction in blood flow when readings are taken from subjects after they have been smoking compared to when they are not.

Smokers are advised to double or treble their intake of Vitamin C since they use many times more than non-smokers. Beta carotene (pro-vitamin A) should also be taken in increased amounts since this acts against singlet oxygen, the most destructive of the many free radicals released by smoking.

American author, Gillian Riley, has written an excellent book on giving up smoking called *How to Stop Smoking and Stay Stopped for Good**.

Cutting Down Drinking

For some it is not possible to cut down – it is better to give up altogether. The problem with drinking is that it puts yet another strain on the liver and other elimination systems and in particular the liver's control and management of cholesterol, a major factor in arterial disease. However, evidence supports the drinking of a small quantity of red wine (say two glasses a day) and there are some indications that an occasional tot of whisky can benefit the

*Vermilion, London 1992.

circulation too. Otherwise spirits are not recommended. Beer drinking is also not recommended because of the high amounts of calories, yeasts and sugars involved.

Dietary Measures

It has been shown that dietary measures are THE controlling factor in the prevention of atherosclerosis, if they are started early enough. If they are not, then they need to be implemented once a course of therapy, such as that described above, has redressed arterial damage to the point where the person can favourably influence their progress (*see Chapter 7*).

Oral Chelation

This is a specific form of nutrition directed at first to complementing the intravenous chelation therapy, and subsequently to maintaining the vitamin/mineral status quo. It is designed to replace any wanted minerals which the therapy may have removed and to provide the body, during the recovery period, with ample stores of protective minerals which are often in short supply in the modern diet, such as magnesium and selenium – the average British diet, for example, does not supply anything like sufficient amounts of these two protective minerals.

Vitamins and trace elements are also given to enhance the metabolism of enzymes in the arterial wall and these will then protect against the atherosclerotic process.

A typical formula for oral chelation is as follows and can be seen to be an extremely comprehensive vitamin/mineral supplement which in fact could be taken all the time, though in lower dosage than the eight tablets daily recommended during the treatment course.

The Arterial Disease Clinic in the UK developed the following formula after lengthy observation of circulatory patients' characteristic needs and deficiencies. It is made up in America – a truly international operation. NB: what is interesting is that the dosages given are expressed in percentages of the US RDAs (official recommended daily allowance figures for vitamins/minerals to maintain health) which yet again indicate the widening gap between what is known by nutritional experts and what is officially recognized.

Eight tablets contain:

Vitamins		Percentage of US RDA
Vitamin A (Palmitate) (Water Dispersible)	10,000 IU†	200
Beta Carotene (Vitamin A Activity)	15,000 IU	300
Vitamin D-3	100 IU	25
Vitamin E (d-alpha Tocopheryl Succinate)	800 IU	2667
Vitamin C (Ascorbic Acid, Corn Free)	3,000 mg	5000
Vitamin B-1 (Thiamine HC1)	100 mg	6660
Vitamin B-2 (Riboflavin)	50 mg	2940
Niacin	40 mg	200
Niacinamide	150 mg	750
Pantothenic Acid (d-Calcium Pantothenate)	500 mg	5000
Vitamin B-6 (Pyridoxine HC1/ Pyridoxal-5-Phosphate Complex)	100 mg	5000
Vitamin B-12 (on Ion Exchange Resin)	100 mcg	1667
Folic acid	800 mcg	200
Biotin	300 mcg	100
Choline Citrate/Bitartrate	150 mg	***
Inositol	100 mg	***
Citrus Bioflavonoid Complex	100 mg	***
PABA (Para-Aminobenzoic Acid)	50 mg	***

Minerals		
Calcium (Citrate & Ascorbate Complex)	500 mg	50
Magnesium (Aspartate & Ascorbate Complex)	500 mg	125
Potassium (Aspartate Complex)	99 mg	***
Zinc (Amino Acid Chelate)	25 mg	166
Copper (Amino Acid Chelate)	2 mg	100
Manganese (Aspartate Complex)	20 mg	***
Iodine (Kelp)	200 mcg	132
Chromium GTF* (organically bound with GTF activity-Low Allergenicity)	200 mcg	***
Selenium (Organic Selenium in Amino Acid Complex & Kelp)	200 mcg	***
Molybdenum (Amino Acid Complex)	100 mcg	***
Vanadium (Amino Acid Chelate)	50 mcg	***
Boron (Aspartate/Citrate Complex)	3 mg	***

Trace Elements (from Sea Vegetation)	approx 100 mcg	***

Others

L-Cysteine HC1/N-Acetyl-L-Cysteine	200 mg	***
DL-Methionine	62.5 mg	***
Glutamic Acid HC1	25 mg	***
Betaine HC1	150 mg	***

In a 500-mg synergistically balanced and formulated base of Lecithin (yielding Phosphatidylcholine, Phosphatidylethanolamine and Phosphatidylinositol) you will get Bromelain (minimum 2000 mcu), Pepsin, Trypsin, Chymotrypsin, L-Carnitine, Coenzyme Q-10/Ubiquinone, Ginkgo Biloba, Polysaccharides, Mucopolysaccharides, Choline Citrate, EDTA, Papain, Cayenne, Chickweed, Hawthorne Berry, Pectin, Mistletoe, Garlic (deodorized), Alfalfa (leaf), Ginger, Pantethine, N-Acetyl-L-Cysteine/L-Cysteine, DL-Methionine and Betaine HCL/Glutamic Acid HCL. It contains no yeast, no wheat, no corn, no soy, no milk, no salt, no sugar, no artificial colouring, preservatives or flavouring.

This impressive supplement is made by Douglas Laboratories in Pittsburgh in Pennsylvania. It gives basically a guideline of what to look for when choosing a supplement with application to circulatory disease. Some of the minor ingredients are herbs which are known to have a beneficial effect on the circulation, such as ginko, hawthorne and mistletoe, and these must be considered optional in the context of a regular supplement (*see Chapter 7*).

Exercise

One of the most powerful tools in the treatment of degenerative disease, experts agree, is regular physical exercise. John Buckley of the Arterial Disease Clinic says: 'The anti-ageing properties of regular exercise are so well-documented that it is superfluous to once again make a case for it. Exercise is essential for maintaining optimum body weight, improving mood, lowering bad blood cholesterol, elevating HDL (good) cholesterol, lowering blood fats, and improving any diabetic condition. We encourage all our patients to exercise, but such programmes must be built up slowly according to the individual's physical condition and under careful medical supervision.'

***US RDA has not been established.
†IUs are measurements based on biological activity.

Aerobic exercise – which simply means getting the heart beating faster for about 20-30 minutes a day – is recommended because the heart, like any other muscle, needs to exercise through its range to maintain performance.

But there is no need to invest in expensive exercise equipment or enrol at the gym, unless desired for company, or to establish a regime – walking briskly is now recognized as one of the best ways of exercising the heart.

The reason for this simple enough regime is that walking sets up a subsidiary blood-pumping action in the foot which assists the circulation of blood. Additionally, walking puts stress on bones and is essential for maintaining bone strength and density. John Buckley says, 'Bones stay fit by working against gravity: you can test this theory by going to bed for a week – use it or lose it.'

The key to exercise is regularity and suggests making a commitment, ideally with a friend, to go for a walk at a certain time at least five days a week. The only reason for joining a health club, in his view, is that in paying to use something one is motivated not to waste the facility. Whatever the choices made, tests have shown that any aerobic exercise programme followed for 20 minutes daily can drop elevated blood sugar levels by 40-50 points within six weeks – this information could be of great value to diabetics who are known to have particularly severe forms of circulatory disease, caused mainly by elevated sugar levels in the boodstream.

Incidentally, squash, and possibly jogging, are now thought to be two of the worst forms of strenuous exercise. These cause blood to be driven too hard through the arterial system and if that blood contains the elements which promote arterial disease, then that process is actually speeded up.

The Female Factor and HRT (*Hormone Replacement Therapy*)
This may be advised for menopausal patients with circulatory problems, as it has a positive effect on calcium metabolism, because it promotes retention of this mineral in the bones, thus affording protection not only from atherosclerosis but also from osteoporosis (*see over*). There are a few women who cannot take it because of contraindicated health conditions.

As a result of the slight risk of taking oestrogen, (which Dr Perry for one believes must be weighed against the advantages), this issue does not currently receive the approval of all chelating physicians, but research at this stage certainly supports those who do believe in it, especially as it may also protect against lipid peroxidation, one of the more violent forms of free-radical damage caused by excess (ionic) iron in the blood.

It is thought that pre-menopausal women suffer less from heart attacks and arterial disease than men, partly because oestrogen protects them and partly because, in menstruating, they lose some iron each month. Certainly it is known that after the menopause statistics for the incidence of heart attacks and arterial disease in women rise to equal that of men.

HRT is also a useful tool (when used in conjunction with chelation therapy) for controlling and preventing osteoporosis. This is a condition from which many older women suffer whereby calcium is leached out of bones making them porous and thus desperately prone to fracture. Nine thousand women die of it in the UK each year (figures correspond throughout the West) and a further 22,000 become permanent invalids.

Before the menopause, oestrogen protects women from suffering from this particular disability, but once oestrogen levels drop, the climate is there for it to begin. This phenomenon is thought to be the main reason why the statistics of women suffering from circulatory diseases catch up with men after the menopause: before then two factors protect them – menstruation (*see above*) and the protection from faulty calcium metabolism by oestrogen. The additional and complementary benefit from EDTA chelation therapy is that in stimulating the parathyroids to store calcium correctly osteoporosis may be prevented to a significant degree. Versions of such measures as those described above are deployed by clinics specializing in circulation disorders and they usually have their own referrals to experts in their area who conduct this vital part of the protocol. There is no point in getting better if measures are not going to be taken to stabilize the improvement. You cannot walk away from your body, and especially not its psychological aspects which can make all the difference between stability and decline.

Support and Treatment Therapies

These are almost too numerous to mention – and becoming more numerous by the day as more and more people jump on the admittedly worthy bandwagon – so take care. Here are some of the better-known options to name a few: Acupuncture; Aromatherapy; Autogenics; Biofeedback; Chiropractic (or Osteopathy and Cranial Osteopathy); Colonic Irrigation/Hydrotherapy; Counselling (and Psychotherapy); Herbalism; Homeopathy; Hydrotherapy; Massage; Naturopathy; Nutritional Therapy; Reflexology; Therapeutic Touch (Healing) and Yoga.

There are many other worthy therapies not mentioned here including a whole category of dance and music and movement therapies and others which involve hobbies such as art or pottery, etc.

The key is to identify what it is that relaxes you – if physical things do it, like massage, then investigate all touch therapies, such as the very effective reflexology (foot massage and treatment of the whole body through zones in the foot), or aromatherapy (massage with essential oils) or just straight massage.

If you suffer joint or back pain or headaches it may be wise to check with a chiropractor or osteopath. If you have suffered during your life from bowel irregularity or discomfort, then consider colonic irrigation or colon cleansing. Treatment of this nature does to the colon what chelation does for the arteries and is therefore extremely complementary to the treatment of circulatory problems.

If you need to talk to somebody, get your head together, try a form of counselling.

Acupuncture is good for balancing body energy, while autogenics or biofeedback can help master stress-related symptoms, such as migraine.

Homeopathy, herbalism or naturopathy can give wonderful support to any physical symptom or condition which has not yet responded to the basic therapies undergone.

How do you find a suitable therapy accessible to you and affordable? Leaf through books in bookshops or write to a health consultant (some work for and write in health magazines) for advice about your specific problem. Never be afraid to ask for help – and when in doubt about the type of therapy, always opt for the therapist who seems to relate best to you.

Chelation can Cure: But Who?

Dr Fritz Schellander says of the treatment: 'I've seen people who've had a lot of chelation therapy and it hasn't done them as much good as usual. I don't know why this minority doesn't respond – I suspect because the deeper issues about their person are not addressed.

'There is always another dimension with the heart. It must never be forgotten that the heart is the core of feeling – every feeling you have is reflected there: fear, fright, ambition, love, sexual arousal...

'We take things to heart. We say these things forgetting that they reflect a reality just as solid as that of an electrocardiogram. In my clinic I sometimes find people with heart disease but little arterial disease – a very different ballgame from those with generalized arterial disease. With isolated heart disease I always consider the feelings, spirit...survival.'

This broad approach, which is pretty general among those who work with chelation therapy, leads other doctors to criticize them because they do not simply deploy one measure to treat their patients – how can they therefore be sure that chelation is the measure which is largely working?

Fritz Schellander's reply to this is: 'a single intervention never works in this complex disease. Unless you get a broad holistic concept you are bound to fail.'

Dr Van Der Schaar says: 'This is always brought against us that we do not use a mono-therapy. That's why we call it a holistic approach. You cannot modify someone's metabolism by just one thing. Dose and formula – both are altered to suit each patient, as are attendant measures.'

CHAPTER SEVEN

DIET, ANTIOXIDANTS AND OTHER NUTRIENTS

NOBEL prize-winning scientist Dr Linus Pauling has made a life-time study of nutrition, in particular the therapeutic properties of Vitamin C, and he said: 'Optimum nutrition is the medicine of the future.'

This not only holds true in the treatment of circulatory disease, but also dozens of studies have shown the protective, and at times, interventive role which nutrition has to play in the minimization of all degenerative disease.

Some studies* have related its combined benefits with EDTA to the circulation: others, such as that of Dr Dean Ornish of the Preventive Medicine Research Institute of Sausalito**, have successfully shown a marked improvement in arterial disease symptoms with combined nutritional measures, exercise programmes and stress control.

Yet others (for example one US study carried out on 87,000 female nurses and 22,000 male doctors on the effects of beta-carotene or pro-vitamin A) have concentrated purely on the action of vitamins to show specific benefits from supplementation in the diet. (In this case reducing the risk of getting CHD by 22 per cent and 25 per cent respectively, as well as reducing risk of cancer.)

There seems little doubt that such measures work: what seems surprising is that we have taken so long to realize that we are what we eat. Possibly the most exciting discovery is not this basic tenet but the fact that vitamins, minerals and amino acids, when taken as

*e.g. that by McDonagh, Rudolph and Cheraskin: 'Effect of EDTA Chelation Therapy plus multivitamin trace mineral supplementation upon vascular dynamics', *Journal of Advancement in Medicine* Spring/Summer 1989.
** *The Lancet*, 21 July, 1990.

medicine (that is not in the strengths or combinations in which they may occur in natural foods but in selective strengthened preparations, called therapeutic dosages), may actually behave as medicines and rid the body of toxic overloads, reduce free radical damage, regulate metabolic disorders such as diabetes, and generally control the process of ageing.

In fact this principle has now become so widely acknowledged that organizations as traditional as MAFF (Ministry of Agriculture, Fisheries and Food) Britain launched a £1.65 million research programme in 1991 devoted to finding out how antioxidant nutrients may protect against various illnesses, such as cardiovascular disease, certain cancers and rheumatoid arthritis. And this is only part of a larger European initiative set up to investigate the role of antioxidants (*see page 139*) in which the catering habits of half a million people will be observed. (NB: it is expected that a high intake of antioxidant-rich foods in the diet such as fruits, fresh vegetables and vegetable oils will be shown to give significant protection).

Dietary and Nutritional Factors in Circulatory Disease

Diet is not synonymous with nutrition. Diet is what we eat, nutrition is the principle of using foods and food supplements to promote health, such as vitamins, minerals or amino acids. Both dietary and nutritional measures can be used in the control and prevention of circulatory disease.

There are those who believe that if we eat the correct diet, we do not need nutritional supplementation and, in an ideal world, were food to be grown naturally and without the interference and constraints of twentieth-century environmental, transport, commercial and pollution problems, they would probably be correct.

Meanwhile, it is better perhaps to be realistic and look at how we can cope with eating well within these constraints, for to do otherwise inevitably means to break regimes when eating out or with others which is self-defeating.

Diets for a healthy heart and arterial system are remarkably consistent with diets for the avoidance of cancer, arthritis or any other degenerative or infectious condition – with certain modifications. In circulatory illnesses, issues which emerge as being of prime importance include controlling one's intake of the following: animal fats and proteins, salt and sugar, processed carbohydrates and of course foods containing calcium (e.g. dairy products, cauliflower, asparagus, and some heavily calcium-ed waters, especially if carbonated).

Diet and Arterial Fat Deposits

For some time now it has been thought that fatty deposits seen in artery walls from about the age of 10 are the result of grossly excessive fat intakes characterized by western diets. (For example, the British diet contains no less than 42 per cent fat. Why? Because fat is cheap, fat is tasty, fat is satisfying as it remains in the stomach for longer than starches and proteins, giving a sense of fullness. Needless to say hidden fats in foods and their equally well-hidden additive chemicals, which improve taste and shelf-life further, remain one of the commercial scandals of our day – together with the vast array of foods containing hidden sugar and salt. These have educated western palates into tastes which are extremely bad for health.)

But fat consumption is not tied up so straightforwardly with cholesterol levels in the blood (known to be tied to heart disease) as was originally thought. Recent research has shown that it is the type of fat consumed rather than (within reason) the quantity, which is connected to both the incidence of coronary thrombosis (clots) and coronary atherosclerosis.

Fat falls into three main categories: saturated, as found in meat, eggs, and dairy products; polyunsaturated, found in most vegetable oils used in cooking and in margarine, and monounsaturated, found in foods such as avocados and olives.

Originally it was thought that people with heart and arterial disease should lower the level of all types of fats in the diet, reducing the proportion to no more than 20 per cent. This makes for a rather unpalatable diet, but on the principle of needs must, many people were advised to follow it.

Recent research reported in the *International Journal of Alternative & Complementary Medicine** by leading nutritional

* December 1993.

expert Dr Melvyn Werbach, author of *Nutritional Influences on Illness*, suggests that while evidence is irrefutable that the eating of *saturated* fats is tied to the incidence both of coronary atheroma and coronary thrombosis, the practice of simply reducing or substituting *polyunsaturated* fats in the diet as many do – such as substituting margarine instead of butter – doesn't always work. However, transferring the fat content of the diet to *mono-unsaturates* does protect one from the above conditions, even if fat intake rises to a more palatable 35 per cent of the diet.

HDL, LDL, and Lipoprotein a

To understand why, it is necessary to look at what happens in the body when fats are ingested. Fats in the body are converted into cholesterol (some remain as triglycerides and the level of these in the blood is equally as indicative of likely arterial disease as is a cholesterol level of over six, of which more later).

Cholesterol, being a fat, is insoluble in a water-based solution such as blood, so to be carried about in the bloodstream it has to be enveloped in a water-soluble protein overcoat, known as a lipoprotein (lipo=fat). There are two main divisions of these: high density lipoproteins (HDLs) and low density lipoproteins (LDLs).

LDLs are deployed by the body to transport cholesterol from the liver to parts of the body where it is needed. HDLs carry excess cholesterol back to the liver, but their primary function is to scavenge excess cholesterol which is left in potentially health-damaging places, such as the artery walls, and transport it back to the liver to be broken down and excreted.

Problems arise when there is a shortage of HDLs to facilitate this cleansing process and, lo and behold, we find that the average western diet is fearfully lacking in foods which facilitate the supply of HDLs like fatty fish, such as mackerel, sardines, herrings, and to a lesser extent tuna and salmon and river trout.

The British diet used to include plentiful supplies of such cheap fish as herrings which were once served fresh: now they're more likely to be canned which affects their efficacy somewhat. Also they have fallen out of favour with the rise of convenience foods and frozen foods for microwave purposes.

There are two levels quoted in blood test results; look for one for HDL and one for LDL. It is ideal if the HDL figure is over 20 per cent of the total.

Other dietary measures for reducing cholesterol include eating less dairy products, fewer eggs (less than four a week) and less shellfish, as well as less meat, except for extremely lean poultry and game.

Eating less saturated fat means being aware of foods in which fat is a hidden or not so hidden constituent, such as sausages, luncheon meat, hamburgers, ice cream, cheese, dairy-based products, cakes and biscuits, etc. and doing away with them before they do away with you! Making this single change will go a long way towards improving arterial symptoms and health in general.

Processed foods contain the worst kind of fat – known in the trade as hydrogenated. These are designed to prolong the shelf-life of food by, quite literally 'holding food together'. Unfortunately, because they are not natural fats they are very poorly digested and may end up not just bonding food but bonding to the walls of arteries. Avoiding them could go a long way towards avoiding fatty deposits.

Despite this caveat in respect to processed fats, the taking of some fatty acids in the diet is essential.

EFAs and Cholesterol

To eat fats in an attempt to reduce them may seem like a contradiction in terms but essential fatty acids (EFAs) are what is needed to restore the balance between HDL and LDL cholesterol: they contain omega 3 which helps to balance cholesterol in the blood. There are two groups of EFAs: the fish oil group which can be taken in tablet form (preferably not cod liver oil which as its name suggests, comes from the liver), and EFAs from seed oils such as sunflower, borage flax and evening primrose. (GLA is the name given to a refined extract of the vital component). Both should be taken and, since they are enriched forms of foods already found in nature, generous amounts are quite safe.

Cholesterol levels can also be lowered naturally by taking garlic (*see the Mediterranean diet, page 113*) and by taking one of the B group of vitamins, such as B3 or niacin which has been widely used in Europe for this purpose for almost four decades. Caution should be exercised, however, as in high doses certain forms of B3 have been seen to affect liver function and nutritional advice is needed.

One form of B3, inositol hexacotinate, is thought not to have these deleterious side effects, yet lowers cholesterol levels efficiently, whilst the inositol part of the compound protects the liver. This is achieved without any of the side effects of straight B3 or indeed of cholesterol-lowering drugs (*see Chapter 3*).

Triglycerides

Some doctors believe that high levels of these in the blood are even more dangerous than high cholesterol levels, as an increased level of these make the blood more viscous and more likely to produce clots which might lodge in narrowed arteries. Although an important energy source, most people eat far too much of them. Two examples are cream and fat on meat.

A number of studies have confirmed the benefits of taking both kinds of EFAs as supplements to the diet. One interesting study by the Medical Research Council in Wales divided men who had already had a heart attack into three groups: one of which was asked to cut down on fat intake, the second to take a high-fibre diet, the third to eat (or take as supplements) oily fish regularly.

Although all three of these measures are known to reduce fat levels in the blood, a third fewer men died of a second heart attack in the fish group after two years than the other two.

Lipoprotein a

This is one form of lipoprotein which is really considered to be *the* LDL particle which is bad news in the arterial disease stakes. In a blood test the level must be under two to feel safe: any more and the potential damage to artery walls is considerable. Protection can be had from all anti-oxidant vitamins and minerals, in particular, vitamins A (beta-carotene form), C, E, and the minerals manganese, zinc, copper, selenium and molybdenum.

If blood levels of this are up, take at LEAST 3g of vitamin C throughout the day (more is better) and at least 400 iu of vitamin E including the d-Alpha tocopherol form, and work slowly up to 600 iu unless advised otherwise.

The amino acid L-Lysine is additionally recommended (by Linus Pauling) because this interferes with the binding of LP(a) to fibrin in the walls of the arteries, so interfering with the build-up of plaque.

Protein

In the 1940s and 1950s, a high protein diet was considered advisable, especially for weight maintenance and physical performance. Many athletes took this diet and many died while training of heart failure, before questions began to be asked.

Now it is acknowledged that a high protein intake (especially of red meats and meat containing iron, as well as of eggs) is a potentially lethal practice for several reasons. Firstly, a high protein diet is low in fibre, which is known to protect from arterial disease. Secondly, it renders the system acidic, which promotes degenerative disease further. Thirdly, it contains iron and too much iron has been shown to be a major factor in promoting free radical damage in sites such as artery walls.

The Protein Equation

The amount of protein needed to sustain cell activity and regeneration differs according to age and activity levels but for a mature adult it can be calculated as 1g (0.03 oz) for every 1kg (2.2lb) body weight.

Obviously growing children, people who play a lot of sport and active young adults need more, but the average person who wants to protect themselves against arterial disease needs very little protein, some 100-150g (4-5oz) per day.

This can be taken as easily through beans, grains or pulses and a little fish as through meat, eggs or cheese. The former have the advantage of being vegetable protein and therefore healthier and purer and they also contain fibre. The purity factor in food is of vital importance today as appallingly resistant strains of bacteria have been found in meat and eggs, to say nothing of added hormones, which animals are fed to improve meat texture.

Fibre and a Healthy Breakfast

It is interesting to note that vegetarians have something like 33 per cent less incidence of arterial disease and coronary heart disease than meat eaters, despite the fact that many have sweet teeth and still indulge in one of the other dietary disasters – eating sugar (which is soon converted to fat and cholesterol).

Books, such as the best-selling *Eight Week Cholesterol Cure* by Robert Kowalski and *The Prittikin Diet*, concentrate on the need for fibre, but in particular it has been discovered that fibre from oats has a tremendous part to play in keeping blood vessels healthy. It is a very simple remedy to take two tablespoons of oat bran in the morning (or other forms of whole oats i.e. containing all the fibre) with unsweetened fruit juice NOT milk in order to secure a major protective influence.

If one or two tablespoons of granular lecithin is added to this mix, you get an added benefit since lecithin is instrumental in keeping fats in suspension where they will not adhere to artery walls. (Check its detergent-like action by putting a spoonful in water and seeing what happens in half an hour or so.) Lecithin should be kept in the freezer and only brought into the refrigerator as needed. Like vitamin E and all nutritional oils (which should be refrigerated not frozen) it goes rancid at room temperature and becomes nutritionally worthless, even deleterious.

Adding a soupçon of powdered ascorbyl palmitate (fat-soluble vitamin A) and even powdered whey or acidophilus complex completes the cocktail which can then be taken at the one meal. (NB: purists say acidophilus should be taken between meals – which with busy lifestyles usually means it is either forgotten or taken sporadically.)

A few millet flakes added to the above gives protein and nutritional elements which improve the condition of hair and nails.

The Fruit Factor

Some people wanting to control cholesterol levels prefer to breakfast entirely on fruit (see Harvey and Marilyn Diamond's *Fit for Life*, Bantam, London, 1987). This is excellent provided fruits are washed, peeled or scrubbed to remove chemical sprays, or are (preferably) organically grown. Fruit should be taken apart from other foods, when digestion of them will be rapid and provide energy within half an hour of consumption.

Fruit juice should be taken pure and not too often as juice sources contain concentrated fruit sugars which can lead to excessive sugar consumption without the benefit of the fruit fibres ingested from whole fruit.

Complex Carbohydrates

These are very satisfying to eat as they do not disappear from the stomach too quickly leaving the eater hungry between meals. Brown rice is a wonder food, as is wholewheat pasta, the friend of those with arterial disease, provided the accompanying sauce is not rich and preferably not too meaty or fishy either (*see Food Combining, below*). Buckwheat and couscous are two other grains worthy of dietary consideration.

Beans (lentils and pulses) require new cooking skills to be learned but have their definite dietary rewards. Some may find them indigestible, though, as they are a mixture of starch and protein. This brings us to a principle which stands all age groups in good stead but especially favours those who have reached middle age – food combining.

Food Combining

Dr William Hay was an American doctor whose ideas, like those of many innovative thinkers, did not meet with widespread favour during his lifetime. Looking to address illness with diet he discovered that the energy used to digest food could be released for body maintenance and life in general if foods were used selectively.

He suggested that since an acid medium was required to digest protein and an alkaline medium was required to digest starch, to combine the two in any meal meant that one type of food waited in the stomach while the other was digested, thus doubling the length of time (and energy required) for the absorption process.

In the resultant Hay diet, no food was banned, just eaten separately. The diagram provides the main guidelines for this weight-reducing principle. For those interested in discovering more about this remarkably simple diet, Doris Grant and Jean Joice's book *Food*

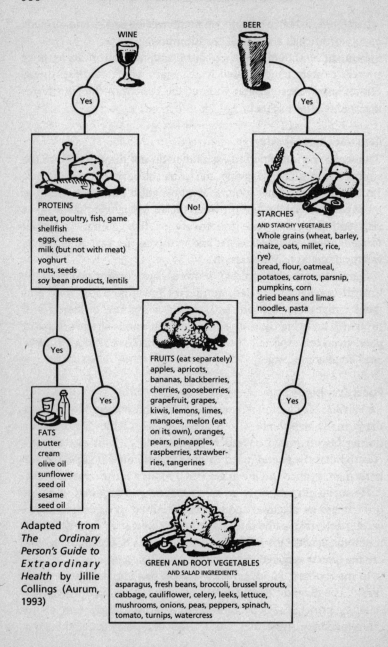

WINE

BEER

Yes

Yes

PROTEINS
meat, poultry, fish, game
shellfish
eggs, cheese
milk (but not with meat)
yoghurt
nuts, seeds
soy bean products, lentils

No!

STARCHES
AND STARCHY VEGETABLES
Whole grains (wheat, barley,
maize, oats, millet, rice,
rye)
bread, flour, oatmeal,
potatoes, carrots, parsnip,
pumpkins, corn
dried beans and limas
noodles, pasta

Yes

Yes

FRUITS (eat separately)
apples, apricots,
bananas, blackberries,
cherries, gooseberries,
grapefruit, grapes,
kiwis, lemons, limes,
mangoes, melon (eat
on its own), oranges,
pears, pineapples,
raspberries, strawber-
ries, tangerines

Yes

FATS
butter
cream
olive oil
sunflower
seed oil
sesame
seed oil

Adapted from
*The Ordinary
Person's Guide to
Extraordinary
Health* by Jillie
Collings (Aurum,
1993)

GREEN AND ROOT VEGETABLES
AND SALAD INGREDIENTS
asparagus, fresh beans, broccoli, brussel sprouts,
cabbage, cauliflower, celery, leeks, lettuce,
mushrooms, onions, peas, peppers, spinach,
tomato, turnips, watercress

*Combining for Health** (with recipes) is recommended. In America this book is also available, and variations of the principle are presented in Harvey and Marilyn Diamond's works.

The Sugar Factor

Professor John Yudkin, a British nutritional expert and author of *Pure, White, and Deadly†* insists that sugar is the primary cause of heart disease. Many people now consume 120lbs of sugar yearly. Those who consume half (still far too high compared to turn-of-the-century consumptions when CHD was virtually unheard of) have six times the chance of coming down with heart disease. Why is this?

Sugar does to the body what aviation fuel would do to a car engine – it burns it out. Natural foods, such as fruits, contain natural sugar bound into their structures, and as such they are released slowly and steadily into the bloodstream; but when refined sugar is consumed, as found in sweets, desserts, chocolates, and fizzy drinks (drinks containing saccharin are just as bad since their taste preserves and encourages the sweet tooth syndrome, quite apart from the fact that artificial sweeteners are chemicals which have been linked to stomach cancer), the body is put on red alert and hormones such as insulin are released into the bloodstream to bring sugar levels back to normal.

Unfortunately this emergency reaction often goes too far the other way, causing blood sugar levels to drop below desired levels, making the person crave a sugar boost all over again. (The same principle occurs with nicotine and smoking.) It is no coincidence that the enormous increase in obesity and diabetes (themselves linked, since obese people often become diabetic) are due to twentieth century per capita sugar consumption going through the roof.

There is an even more sinister link between sugar consumption and peripheral arterial disease which can be brought on by constant distortion of the sugar balance in the blood. Peripheral artery disease can lead to gangrene.

It is important to reduce sugar consumption to the minimum. At first this will be difficult, but it is amazing how quickly the palate

* Thorsons, London, 1984.
† Penguin, London, 1988.

becomes re-educated so that the accidental addition of sugar in tea or coffee as before becomes completely unacceptable.

Salt

Salt is another tasty hidden additive in commercial foods such as soups, casseroles, and ready-prepared freezer and microwave foods. Patrick Holford of the Institute of Optimum Nutrition in London (ION) has said in his excellent little book, *Super Nutrition for Healthy Hearts** that the average person consumes more than 10g of salt a day which is 20 times what we need.

Salt and high blood pressure are linked, as salt causes retention of fluid in the bloodstream. This raises blood volume and blood pressure. (NB: taking water pills, or diuretics, to solve this fluid problem results in the ingesting of a chemical which leaches out valued mineral sources, quite apart from distorting kidney function. Unless the condition is extreme, there are natural diuretics such as B6, dandelion 'tea', etc, which may be implemented – any good herbalist will help with this problem.)

Stimulants such as Tea, Coffee and Other

Stimulants are ageing since they set up an energy overdraft situation in the body bank, drawing on energy reserves which would otherwise be devoted to valuable, even life-saving repair work to body tissues, such as the arterial system.

This is a 'play-now, pay-later' policy which unless balanced by compensatory periods of rest and relaxation will lead to some form of degenerative disease.

Dairy is Dire

The single action of cutting dairy products out (or dramatically down) could of itself go a long way towards redressing the degeneration of arteries. This means less or no milk, cheese, cream, cream cheese, most yoghurt, and last but by no means least, butter. However, a word about butter, or rather about its rival, margarine.

Butter is far better for you than margarine. Margarine is produced from seeds which are processed to within an inch of their

*ION Press, London, 1989.

natural lives. Apart from being heated (even so-called cold-pressed margarines like safflower have to rise in temperature to 45° C) the numerous chemical processes used to purify, process and 'butter' the taste inevitably result in additives being present which no body needs. As Doris Grant says in her excellent book, 'butter is better' and she devotes a chapter to why.

A small pat of butter a day will not harm, but it is preferable to substitute pure virgin olive oil wherever possible, such as in salad dressings and for frying food (a bad habit in itself). Oil must be cold-pressed and kept cool at all times. Again it is a question of acquired taste, but it is a taste that is well worth developing, because olive oil actually helps the body to deal with unwanted levels of saturated fats.

The Mediterranean Diet

Curious researchers, noting how much olive oil, red wine, garlic and salads the French (and for that matter the Italians and Spanish) consumed and how low, compared to Britain and USA, was their incidence of heart disease, discovered that all of these foods protected from cardiovascular conditions. Red wine contains certain protective ingredients which promote arterial health, provided it is drunk in moderation (no more than half a bottle a day of GOOD red wine, not a cheap one which will be full of additives).

Garlic

Garlic is now an object of research supported by the British Heart Foundation, which has recently funded a £24,000 trial at the John Radcliffe Infirmary in Oxford to study its anti-cholesterol properties. Its other healing properties suggest that *allium sativum* is one of the most powerful medicinal herbs known. Researchers in Germany, the USA and Britain have recently confirmed its ability to regulate blood pressure, reduce high cholesterol and lipid levels, improve blood circulation and fight infections.

Nutrition for Healthy Arteries: Prevention in a Pill

Many nutritional supplements today are being marketed as antioxidants. This is because report after report has confirmed their beneficial effects on everything from IQ levels, antisocial behaviour and delinquency in the young to age-associated problems such as arthritis, high blood pressure, high cholesterol levels and general debility.

The term anti-oxidant refers to the facility of certain vitamins and minerals to protect the body from the oxidizing effect of free radicals, the effect in the body being similar to that observed when opened wine goes sour or butter goes rancid. Leaving leather goods out in the sun is another example – the cross-linking of the fibres which occurs in the presence of air and sunlight resembles very closely what happens to skin when it 'leathers' and wrinkles from too much exposure to the sun and elements. Obviously if this kind of effect happens inside the body it is responsible for tissues hardening and becoming less supple as is characterized by ageing.

Vitamins both arrest and slow down this process, particularly vitamins with strong antioxidant properties, such as vitamins A, C, E and certain minerals, such as chromium, magnesium, zinc and selenium. All vitamins and all minerals play key roles in the body, but some are indispensable. It is highly significant that at least two of the most indispensable of the minerals, especially in view of their advantageous effect on normalizing blood pressure and heart action and general antioxidant effects respectively, are magnesium and selenium, both of which are in short supply in the British diet (and probably elsewhere).

Selenium is depleted because the soils in which crops are grown now lack this vital trace mineral. Low selenium levels are linked to coronary artery disease.

Magnesium is depleted because of the British habit of eating over-refined food. White flour has lost 82 per cent of the magnesium content found in whole grain and white sugar has lost 99 per cent of the magnesium found in molasses and brown sugar is little better.

Factors such as these ensure that the average British diet provides just under 250mg magnesium a day which is about half what should be taken. (US RDA figures recommend 350-400mg per day and these are thought to be characteristically low, as most RDAs are.)

Magnesium works in apposition to calcium to balance the electrical charges in the cell. Michael Murray, ND and Joseph Pizzoro,

ND who have written a definitive work called *The Encyclopaedia of Natural Medicine**, write: 'An intracellular deficiency of free magnesium is a major etiological factor in hypertension, as its levels are consistently low in hypertensives as compared with nomotensives (those with normal blood pressure). In one double-blind clinical study magnesium supplementation lowered low blood pressure by 12/8mm mercury in 19 out of 20 subjects in the experimental group, compared to none 0/4 in the placebo group.'

However, before rushing out to buy supplements, be aware that some (cheaper) forms of magnesium (inorganic) are poorly absorbed and it is best to buy supplements that consist largely of magnesium citrate, orotate, aspartate, that is in its organic form.

Vitamins and Minerals: What to Choose and What Dosage

The above advice brings to light one of the major problems with vitamin and mineral supplementation – what to choose? In a society which now recognizes that vitamins, minerals and amino acids have a valuable role to play in health, there are precious few nutritional experts to give advice on personal data, such as hair analysis, blood profile, etc.

Beware of believing that being a doctor qualifies someone to give such advice – the medical syllabus provides virtually no information about nutritional matters except where they become medically diagnosable and treatable, such as with scurvy (the clinical lack of vitamin C). For every person who reaches that extreme there are probably a million who are vitamin C deficient in some level or another.

Most people get by on a vitamin/mineral composite daily tablet, but with arterial disease this, while helpful, is not enough. More specific supplementation is necessary; supplementation which, ideally, is tailored to personal profiles such as blood analysis or those designed by a nutritional expert.

A Word about Antioxidants

'A' vitamins consist of two main groupings, retinol which is fat

* Macdonald Optima, London 1990.

soluble and therefore stored in the body, so some caution in dosage must be acknowledged (thought not as much as was originally thought), and beta carotene, research into which was mentioned previously (*see page 101*). This wonder vitamin does not hold the overdose dangers of retinol, as the body only converts it as needed and research has shown that it has considerable protective benefits to offer from all forms of degenerative disease. Make sure it is taken in its natural form – often produced from the algae Dunaliella.

'*B*' *vitamins* are a special case. They help with stress and three of them, in particular B1, B3, and B6, have positive effects on the circulation. Since 1984, Dr Stephen Davies, a medical nutritional expert, has assessed the nutritional status of some thousands of his patients. His measurements have included vitamin levels, trace and toxic metal levels. More than seven out of every 10 people tested were borderline or severely deficient in B vitamins. Since toxicity is known to accumulate with age it affords an added reason for taking antioxidants to minimize this damage.

B6 is a mind diuretic and can be used to supplement (or hopefully replace after treatment with EDTA) the use of chemical diuretics. B3 lowers blood cholesterol levels (*see above*) and B1 helps mood, as well as facilitating the processing of alcohol in the liver.

Vitamin 'C' is possibly the most important antioxidant vitamin of all. Linus Pauling has been largely responsible for making the scientific world aware that vitamin C taken in sufficient quantities is a superb free-radical mopper. It fights infection and combats degeneration.

Recent research by the UCLA in California has demonstrated that men taking more than 400mg of vitamin C a day cut their risk of heart disease almost in half, compared to men taking only 100mg or less. This is of great interest in respect to contentions by health authorities that RDAs are sufficient to maintain health.

Comparative studies with animals who can make their own vitamin C (a facility man has lost) reveal that they make the equivalent of 1,000 to 20,000 mg per day for their uses. The average diet is lucky to contain 100-200 mg of this precious vitamin. (NB: drinkers of orange juice, who believe they are getting enough vitamin C, should know that research has shown that commercially grown oranges can, and often do, contain *none* of this vitamin by the time they are eaten.)

Suffice it to say that this vitamin should be taken on a regular daily basis in far greater quantities than is normally practised. Most people above middle age can safely and sensibly take 3-5g throughout the day – if the bowel becomes loose ease back the dosage until it has stabilized.

Vitamin E is so important in the protection of the cardiovascular system that blood tests usually list its value. This is no doubt a reflection of the fact that low serum E levels are strongly related to heart disease. Ideally the blood level should be over 19. Any lower and supplementation is vital. Most heart sufferers are advised to take therapeutic dosages of at least 400 iu a day, working up slowly to 600-800 iu. NB: vitamin E has an anti-coagulant effect so this must be taken into account if anticoagulants are being taken, otherwise blood-clotting time can be delayed beyond levels that are safe. However vitamin E is a much better anticoagulant to take than drugs.

Vitamin E works in conjunction with vitamin C to provide protection against free radical activity.

'*Co-Q-10*' or *Co-enzyme-Q-10*, was isolated in the mid-1950s and since then has shot to nutritional 'fame' for its key role in the production of energy in the cells. Unfortunately, like so many vital body secretions and enzymes, production slows down in middle age and we suffer progressively from its deficit. Metabolic studies have demonstrated that CoQ10 plays a vital role in the utilization of oxygen by the cells and is, therefore, essential for the health of all human tissues and organs. But its effects have been seen to relate particularly to the heart. When 60mg a day of CoQ10 were given to 25 hypertensive patients for eight weeks, there was a significant decrease in blood pressure. Fifty-four per cent of the patients had a mean blood pressure fall greater than 10 per cent.

In Japan more than 14 million people take CoQ10, which is hardly surprising when it is noted that it also helps with diseases such as diabetes, angina pectoris, congestive heart failure and peridontal disease.

It is of grave import to note that some are known to inhibit the production and action of CoQ10 in the tissues. If this medication is taken it should at least be combated by taking additional CoQ10 as well.

Amino Acids

These are the latest to arrive on the supplement chain and much is still being learned about them. Suffice it to say, they are the building blocks of the body, derived from proteins, but an ample supply of proteins in the diet does not necessarily protect one from shortages as their construction in the body relies on complex metabolic steps which may or may not be completed in a state of illness.

Thus a general amino acid supplement is not a bad thing to take on a daily basis. Linda Lazarides advises taking L-Lysine for angina but points out that as much as 6,000mg a day may have to be taken. Once again we are confronted with the possibility of imbalance if one is taken in great excess to another, so an overall supplement of aminos, plus extra Lysine may be advised. Some aminos need to be taken on an empty stomach to be effective – again advice is needed.

Lazarides also advises taking EFAs, but warns that once again those on blood thinners will have to proceed with caution, taking the lower dose recommended on the packaging until advised.

Here are some points worth noting:

- Take NO vitamins or minerals with tea, coffee or alcohol – their effect will block absorption
- Take zinc separately from other minerals, if possible
- Take organic forms of minerals, not inorganic, chelated if possible
- Order regular fresh supplies of supplements (especially oil-based) rather than stockpiling large sizes which may 'go off'
- NEVER take supplements with iced water or drink – this impairs their absorption
- Consider taking a digestive aid, such as Pineapple Bromelaine or (especially if you are acid deficient, which people over forty may be) Betaine Hydrochloride

John Stirling of Biocare UK Ltd, who specializes in enzyme preparations (the supplementation of the future), believes that unless good food and nutrients are digested there is no point in taking them. One of the major problems with degenerative diseases is that absorption is impaired and this deficiency must be helped until the system reaches a better level of homeostasis.

In addition, it is wise to take a good acidophilus supplement to aid and balance digestively helpful gut flora, as with increasing age intestinal flora becomes compromised by antibiotics taken in the past, and which are still being ingested unknowingly in food and water supplies, and by chemicals in packaged and preserved foods and household cleaning agents, etc, and by chemicals in fuels and in the atmosphere.

Summary of Categories of Nutritional Supplements for a Healthy Heart and Circulatory System

- ❧ Vitamin/mineral supplement containing antioxidants mentioned above and a good supply of magnesium
- ❧ EFAs
- ❧ Amino acid supplement
- ❧ Lecithin (or Phosphatidyl Choline)
- ❧ CO-Q-10
- ❧ Digestive enzymes such as Pineapple Bromelain or Betaine HCL
- ❧ Live acidophilus supplement
- ❧ Bifido Growth Factor

Herbs and Other Circulatory Aids

Ginko Biloba

Ginko Biloba is often cultivated as an ornamental tree in streets and parks throughout the world for its beauty and long life. It is resistant to the pollution often found in big cities. This is hardly surprising when it is discovered that the plant has long been part of the traditional Chinese pharmacopoeia, being first cited as a medicinal agent more than 5,000 years ago, when it was known as the plant of youth for its general tonic properties.

To this day, in China, people inhale decoctions of the leaves to alleviate asthma and bronchitis, where it is known to be beneficial for the heart and lungs.

A systematic study of the plant was initiated in Europe around 1960 after several newspapers had reported that Mao Tse Tung had been greatly helped by it. Allowing for its extremely low toxidity, the extract was tested for its ability to improve central and peripheral circulatory disorders. It proved to increase blood flow in a large number of diseases related to depleted circulation, especially in the brain and lower limbs. With this sort of record, and its harmlessness, it is certainly worth a month's try.

Other herbs which are known to have significant effects on various aspects of cardiovascular disease are: hawthorn berries, lily of the valley, broom, lime blossom, valerian, mistletoe and yarrow. To employ these, it is necessary to find a qualified herbalist who will utilize very great skills in treating aspects of this disease safely.

Herbalists, nutritional experts etc can usually be located by reading advertisements in local health publications or by writing to the publication for advice. Local health centres may help, as may health food shops. Some public libraries carry lists. Word of mouth is the best recommendation, but remember that what helped your colleague (even with the same condition) may not necessarily help you. Trial and error is the only way – your good health the goal. Never stay with a therapist you don't like or respect or completely trust.

Overview of Diet and Nutrition

It is not the purpose of this book to give specific dietary and nutritional advice, because it is important for each person to realize how specific their needs are, tied in as they are to eating habits, work schedules, physical activities, age, sex, health, emotional life and family relationships, etc.

In the very near future it will be considered as necessary to visit one's nutritional advisor as it is to visit one's dentist. Suffice it to say, it could be a very good investment to seek advice of this kind if circulatory disease exists (*see Useful Addresses*).

CHAPTER EIGHT

CASE HISTORIES AND COMMENT

PRESENTING case histories to illustrate and support the cause of a major therapy which has not yet been generally accepted is a responsibility which requires diligent research, not just for supportive evidence but also for its counterpart.

During 1987-8, while considering the subject of chelation for inclusion in the fortnightly alternative health column I then wrote for the *Guardian*, I tried to find people who had had negative experiences. The fact that they were not to be found I attributed as much to early cases being *in extremis* with their circulatory condition, and therefore well pleased with any results they received than to the success of the treatment – after all the first clinic in London had only opened in 1985, and they and their patients were still finding their way.

However, continued evidence of patients' general experience of abatement in physical symptoms, such as claudication, angina, breathlessness, TIAs (Transient Ischaemic Attacks – little strokes), cold extremities, sight and hearing problems, varicose vein ulcers, gingivitis, diabetes/demand for insulin, etc, suggested it was the therapy that was working rather than their pressing need for it. That it was working *in extremis* made it all the more remarkable. Furthermore, improvements often continued for months or years after the treatment course had ended.

During, or soon after, the treatment people found they could run for the bus when they could not walk more than a few steps before: they could lower their drug dosage and sometimes come off supportive medication altogether. In general they spoke in glowing terms of how they could now get on with their lives.

High blood pressure was one symptom which almost generally

abated, sometimes to normal levels. Since high blood pressure damages artery walls, stresses the heart and exacerbates arterial disease this was significant.

In 1994, researching for this book, I spoke to some of the patients that I had spoken to before. An overview was emerging of feelings of general wellbeing and homeostasis (that is, health remaining stable), but did they need further treatment? Some did, some didn't – it varied.

In Holland, the most senior of all the European chelating physicians, Professor Van Der Schaar (since 1979 he has given over 110,000 treatments to over 5,000 patients), gave his professional opinion that a treatment every 17 days was the ideal mode for those with established or advanced arterial disease. In London, pioneer patient, Valerie Tomkins, said she had settled on a maintenance programme of one treatment about every six weeks. In her seventies now, she is typical of patients having chelation therapy for whom it is not surprising that they will have to work harder to maintain homeostasis than people in their forties and fifties with little disease.

There are however a number of patients who seem to be able to change and adapt their lifestyle sufficiently not to need top-ups at all, or only sporadically. Valerie Tomkins admits she has a stressful family life which has persisted since her heart attack in 1983.

Towards Homeostasis

The re-establishing of homeostasis after treatment is an attainable ideal, noted by cardiac experts such as Professor Vincent (*see Chapter 5*) who also sees its reverse more often in operation in sick patients: 'In medicine the idea of vicious circles is true. You take heart failure. If the heart fails to pump blood well enough in one beat then a bit of blood accumulates. Next time it's a bit overfilled so a bit less efficient. In heart failure there's a spiralling down which requires a lot of therapy until you get back up to a particular point and then it can be held. Tucked back in there is a mechanism which you push back into balance of operation and then it's maintained in spite of the fact that the treatment is no longer there.'

This is what seems to happen to the patients who have chelation therapy. They no longer need their drugs, props, and restricted lifestyles: their fear of overdoing things abates and they are re-empowered to take charge of their health instead of their sickness taking charge of them.

Four Case Histories

Case history: V. T. (woman – aged 72).
I had my first heart attack while in Spain on holiday [this is a common pattern – why do we get sick on holiday?] After a few days' rest I got myself home, went straight to bed and called the doctor. He thought I'd had an 'oesophageal event' and dismissed me, but I was dissatisfied and took myself to have a complete check up at BUPA [UK providers of private medical insurance and diagnostic services].

The ECG showed I'd had a heart attack. They also discovered that I had very high blood pressure. I was treated for the high blood pressure but nothing further was suggested and I realized this was just controlling symptoms, not addressing my problems, so I began to read up about my condition.

I read books and articles about chelation therapy from the US and could see the feasibility of such a treatment but nobody was doing it in the UK. Then James Kavanagh [the original director of the London Chelation Clinic] turned up. He had been to Holland to study the techniques from Van Der Schaar and in 1985 opened a small clinic in the corner of another clinic in Harley House [in London].

I plucked up the courage and signed up for 20 treatments. My friend came too for moral support – he didn't need the treatment as I did but he said he felt much better after it and his hair improved.

I wanted to know what one did next. The doctor [Perry] never pushed me. I even wondered if he believed in it! Anyway I decided to have another 10. This year (1994) I decided to have one every six weeks – the treatment takes effect for six weeks after you've stopped so it made sense to have another after that interval.

I've had all the tests before and after – blood tests, uroanalysis, Doppler [*see Chapter 3*] – and from my first Doppler to the one I had last week I have consistently improved: all my figures have gone down.

I admit I have never regularly taken the oral chelation tablets they give you, and never the dose they recommend, nonetheless my hair and blood analysis (which I have done independently from a nutritional expert) reveal my mineral status is nearly perfect.

The only adverse effect I get is I get a bit tired the day after an infusion – didn't used to but I'm 72 now. At one stage during a course of treatment I had cystitis twice. I tended to get 24 hours of sensitivity after the treatment. Dr Perry did all the checks and said he didn't think it was the treatment and what else was I doing? Well, I was swimming daily in highly chlorinated pool and was also bathing daily with essential oils. I stopped first the essential oils in the bath water and then left the swimming pool – I never had any more problems after that.

My GP doesn't know I'm doing it [the treatment]. My heart specialist originally said, 'Don't touch chelation, it won't do you any good.' Yet he confirms I've regained heart muscle and am doing very well.

NB: The right of patients to choose (or deny) themselves treatment must always be preserved and is reflected in the *Patients' Charter*, a copy of which is available to anyone and can usually be collected at local council buildings.

Case History: RC, (Male – upper middle age)
My first heart attack must have occurred when I was on holiday staying in France in 1987. I kept getting this severe pain in the upper back. Thought I'd slipped a disc. But I would wake up in the night with it and any exertion like packing up the car made it worse. I discussed with my wife whether the coffee and French pastries might be contributing to the pain and I stopped them and through cutting out tea, coffee and pastries I did improve but not much.

On my return to England I had to go to the bank – I wanted a business loan so I had to have a medical checkup. The doctor there discovered I had high blood pressure, 190/90 but apart from that he said I was fine. I decided to cut out fats and transform my diet and my blood pressure dropped to 130/70 and has stayed there ever since.

But I still had angina. I decided to have a checkup with a cardiologist associated with a leading London hospital. In October 1988 I had a treadmill test and was told 'there is nothing you can do really'. I asked about diet and was told 'eat what you like'. I was mad about this because I knew diet had helped me before. He [the specialist] also told me I didn't need to exercise – a warm bath was all I needed.

I began to have more problems. I spoke to a friend who worked in another London hospital, she arranged for me to see the Professor of Cardiology there. That was June 1989. He diagnosed a 90 per cent blockage in my coronary arteries and suggested angioplasty. I went in on Wednesday, was done on Thursday, came out Saturday with drug treatment.

In the following year, I was carrying a bag of waste to the dustbin when I felt queer. I went to my GP who confirmed I was having a heart attack and must be conducted urgently to hospital. It had to be the original London hospital in my area. Once there, a doctor looked at me and said I could go home: 'you look perfectly all right to me'. My wife refused. If she had not been so adamant I would not be here now because I had a severe heart attack that night.

It was a horrendous experience. I was put in a room with three other patients on life support machines, two of which died, one had his family screaming around him. There they were, screaming and shouting right next to the intensive care unit for heart patients.

My attack started at 9.00 p.m. and I was in agony. They tried to find the registrar. At midnight they got hold of him and he gave me a streptokinase injection and immediately the pain started to ease. Apparently that dissolves blood clots.

The next day the original consultant cardiologist turned

up. He said, 'that shot we gave you cost £750. We only had two in the hospital and you got one.'

I later found out that up in Scotland doctors carry this around normally. I was truly shocked that a major hospital in London only had two shots.

After three sleepless nights, following transferral to a general ward through which ambulance crews were trundling people all night with doors crashing, and the TV on all night, I started another heart attack. I insisted my wife help move me out and I did move to a second hospital. They gave me another balloon angioplasty at 3.00 a.m. As I was being wheeled out of the theatre the surgeon said, 'It was a great success.'

Great success? I thought. I am still lying here in such terrible pain I can't move and you tell me that?

After I was discharged on three drugs, I felt better for about two months. Then I started to feel unwell again, so unwell I was spending two to three days in bed each week.

One day my wife said, 'Get out of bed, you are fading away. I won't let this happen. We have heard about this treatment [chelation] and you are having it.'

In April '91 I went to see Wayne [Dr Perry]. It was the best day's work I ever did. I had a Doppler. One carotid artery [leading to the head] was 70 per cent blocked. On one artery they couldn't get a reading because there was too much disturbance.

After 20 treatments I felt great. I had bought a complete kitchen which I was going to fit, but I delayed when I started feeling ill. After the treatment my wife said you couldn't knock me down. I laid the ceramic tiled floor, my wife mixed the cement. I was so fit I dug the garden over. The difference was unbelievable. My carotid blockage was reduced by 30 per cent.

Through all this I kept my GP informed. He was in accord with my trying the treatment. When I later had a checkup with the senior cardiologist at the hospital (he has some post in Europe too), I asked him about chelation to see what he'd say and he said, 'Don't touch it, it doesn't work.'

I have now had 30 treatments and, after meeting a patient in the clinic who was having the treatment on the National Health [a pioneering step], I asked my doctor to write to the heart specialist to see if I could have it too. When I next saw him I knew he'd received the letter but he had six senior doctors around him and he never raised it and neither did I, to spare his feelings.

He did tell me I was down for a triple bypass and I asked him what protection it gave me from further heart attacks. 'Oh it won't stop you from having another heart attack,' he said. 'How reassuring,' I thought. 'Here I am about to have another heart operation and I'm told it mightn't work.'

It reminded me of a remark I'd heard in the arterial clinic. Three farmers had come in from Kenya. They did have a chelation clinic in Kenya, but local medicos got it closed down. One very fit man had gone to his doctor and the doctor had said, 'Why don't you have a bypass?' 'Do I need it?' he had asked. 'No,' the doctor said, 'but it would give you another ten years of life.' He said he then decided to hot foot it to the UK to have chelation therapy instead.

RC is now fit and active. His wife and he both follow a carefully controlled diet low in fat, meat and dairy foods and high in fibre and fresh fruit and vegetable content. His wife once followed a diet consisting entirely of grapes for a month. She had so much energy she used to spring out of bed singing in the mornings, to such an extent her husband begged her to 'tone it down'.

What seems disturbing about this case history is the picture it paints about lack of peace and quiet in intensive care in a leading London teaching hospital. As RC says: 'How do they expect patients to get better if they can't sleep for noise and commotion?' Also disrupting to patient welfare were the battles RC and his wife had to fight on his account to get the treatment he wanted at the very time when he should have been surrendering to recovery.

The general criticism of chelation therapy – it doesn't work (*see* Chapter 5) was again in evidence.

Case History: ET (male – 74)

I had my first heart attack at 45, a minor affair. But I viewed it as a warning and transferred my job from the Inland Revenue to Customs in Portsmouth. I'd only been there six months when I had another heart attack, a sharpish one. They wanted me to retire then – at 46!

After that there were serious constraints on what I did. I was cossetted, could drive the car a bit, couldn't do a lot more. I had learned pottery earlier so I took that up again, exhibited a bit. I think you could say I was fairly active in some ways, in others not. Then I had another scare while on holiday in France and after that I had an angiogram. It was discovered then that I couldn't have a bypass, the damage to my coronary arteries was too messy.

I began to sink then, lost hope. I was 67 and didn't expect to see 70. I was sleeping a lot, no energy – I knew I was dying. My wife said I was getting fuzzy and forgetful. Then in April 1988 I read the article in the *Guardian* about chelation therapy. I went to my doctor immediately who said, 'Why not? We can't do any more for you.'

After two or three chelations, I saw a sharpening of my mind and then after 16 or 17 I noticed an enormous difference and so did my friends. My wife said it was like a miracle. Before that I could only walk 200-300 yards and now I could walk two or three miles.

Since then I've done a lot more pottery, and I also teach it once a week. I love that. I sporadically have top up treatments but it's difficult as I live on the Isle of Wight. I'm coming up to 74 this summer and am getting a bit more angina than I did soon after the treatment. My carotids are not responding as well as we would like them to, but my doctor advised against carotid angioplasty, the medical alternative, as it might cause more problems than it would cure if a bit of plaque broke off and went somewhere else. My cholesterol level is now very good, 4.6.

I know I'm getting a bit older now and not so fit as before but I've had some more very good years when I was able to be useful and I shall forever be grateful for that article in the *Guardian*. At the time it saved my life.

Case History: Mr S. (Male – aged 56, a diabetic since 1988)
I was taking 12 National Health prescribed drugs when I first came to the clinic in July 1993 – now reduced (early 1994) to six a day. Also my insulin intake has been reduced by two-thirds.

In July '93 when I started, I was struggling to walk on level ground for more than four or five minutes: now I can walk four or five times as far. I have no chest pains any more [he suffered badly from angina], but I still get cramp in the back of my legs, though they're much better than before.

When I first visited the clinic I was sceptical, so I had a good look round before deciding to shell out a couple of thousand quid. But now I've had 20 chelation treatments with them (between 29 July 1993 and 8 December 1993) – one a week.

I got relief after the fourth or fifth week when I suddenly felt quite a bit of improvement. I came home on the Wednesday and on the Friday I suddenly found myself doing something I hadn't done for 12 months. The improvement came just as quick as that. It was the breathlessness which had got me down before; it happened when I did anything physical at all.

By Christmas last year I was feeling better than I've felt for two or three years and my tests show I've had 20 per cent overall improvement in my arteries.

In 1986 I'd had balloon angioplasty on my worst (left) leg which had gone numb and it did help for a time. But then they did nothing except give me tablets until March '93 when they tried to do an angiogram. By that time my leg arteries were so blocked up again they couldn't get the wires up and they dismissed me, said they couldn't treat me. They also abandoned any idea of doing a bypass operation, which they had considered for my angina.

Why did they wait all those years from the time of the first treatment? By that time I was beyond help.

It was at that point that a friend of mine, a medical journalist, told me about chelation therapy. I then went to my GP who admitted he knew nothing about it but said, 'What have you got to lose? They're offering you nothing.'

When I came to the clinic I saw there were patients getting treatment on the national health so I went to my doctor again and he wrote a letter. Then began another saga.

The local health authority refused the doctor's request and repeated there was nothing more they could do. I decided to take it further, wrote to my MP and eventually drew his attention to the health minister's commitment [in June 1992, *see page 136*] to allow chelation therapy on the National Health provided it was considered suitable by the consulting doctor.

My doctor did agree, but the local health authority turned me down. They said they were considering chelation therapy but at this stage could not allow it. I then wrote again to my MP, who wrote on my behalf to the National Health Authority. They wrote back saying that whilst chelation therapy was available within the National Health for some conditions, it was not considered to be effective for cardiovascular diseases and therefore they disallowed my request. I'm still in the process of fighting this and I won't give up.

Chelation and Establishment Approval

Wherever one turns – America, Canada, Kenya, Britain – there is a struggle to get this 30-year established treatment accepted by either government health schemes or private insurance companies – companies who are quite prepared to pay for a treatment such as bypass surgery which will cost them on average ten times more than a course of chelation. What deters them?

The *safety* of chelation therapy is not in question. That has been established by long experience with treatments for which EDTA is accepted protocol, such as a blood condition known as thalassaemia, or for heavy metal poisoning.

What is not proved to medical requirements (double-blind trials) is its efficacy in treating circulatory disease. However, there have been some 200 scientific studies concentrating on the specific effects of EDTA in circulatory disease (more than have ever been done, as stated earlier, in respect to the medical procedures of bypass surgery and angioplasty) and these, plus overwhelmingly positive empirical evidence, must surely present sufficient grounds for experimental use in certain areas.

For example, what about those medicines that can't help any more? Those patients whom the medical profession calls by the rather besmirching term of 'refractory'? Since chelation is safe and they have been given up anyway what have they – or anyone else – to lose?

Chelation v. Leg Amputation

There is one particular group of patients, those suffering from peripheral ischaemia (starvation of blood to extremities such as legs) who would surely be ideal as pilot groups for the study of the efficacy of chelation.

According to a report in *The Lancet* (Vol 339 April 11, 1992) between 500 to 1,000 people per million of the population in western Europe suffer each year from critical ischaemia and as many as a quarter of these are faced with major amputations.

The medical joke about having your leg off becomes a grim reality for 6,000 to 10,000 people each year, and although bypass surgery can be effected on femoral (leg arteries) it is a longer and more difficult operation than amputation (up to 8 hours of a surgeon's time rather than a mere half hour for amputation). Furthermore, says *The Lancet*, the former technique 'commits the surgeon to long-term responsibilities' whereas with amputation 'the surgeon can quickly dissolve responsibility to the limb fitter and rehabilitation specialist.'

It is not difficult to envisage which option is likely to be more often recommended to the patient when busy National Health surgeons are involved, bearing in mind that balloon angioplasty (the other alternative) may be effective but is unlikely to last.

Surely if these people knew about the option of chelating they would opt for it every time over surgery, even if the treatment carried a risk, which it doesn't unless kidney function is seriously impaired.

In fact, there have been research projects proferred to chelating physicians in America: first they must concede that one leg be removed by surgery and then they may treat the other by chelation. In one such case, where the surgeon inadvertently cut off the better of a patient's two legs (the other was subsequently saved by chelation) the patient is suing the surgeon.

This circumstance is apparently ideal for comparing two treatments and their efficacy for trial purposes, but leads to a fundamental question of ethics. Is the pursual of scientific proof interfering with the way patients are sometimes regarded and treated?

Case history patients who had had bypass surgery and angioplasty before chelation therapy sometimes complained of this: that they had been made to feel more like guinea pigs than patients and furthermore that they had not always been acquainted with the risks of any surgical procedure they were about to undergo, nor what the consequences might be. Some had actually been frightened into taking decisions regarding surgery on an 'or else' basis (this factor is more generally in evidence with private patients).

One patient showed me a letter from his cardiac physician after he refused to take beta blockers as recommended. 'I will not be held responsible for what happens to you,' the letter said tersely. To be fair: consultants are probably exasperated into such responses by some of their patients who expect to be 'got better' by drugs or surgery while they still carry on as before, eating the wrong things, drinking, smoking, etc.

Nonetheless, patient consideration does seem to have gone out of the more commercial end of the cardiovascular branch of medicine, especially in America. Chelating physicians as a bunch seem to take far more joy in their medicine than the average specialist, probably because they are confronted with very sick people who get better and stay better.

'Our first duty is to support and comfort the patient.' Dr Wayne Perry of the Arterial Disease Clinic in London says. 'Our aim must always be to empower patients, not disempower them,' says Dr Fritz Schellander of the Liongate Chelation Clinic in Tunbridge Wells. 'The doctor's first aim is not to harm,' says Dr Van Der

Schaar of the Leende Chelation Clinic near Eindhoven in the Netherlands.

EDTA Chelation Therapy, Oxygen/Ozone Therapy, therapies for help in stress management, advice on diet and lifestyle changes are all empowering measures. The patient feels better, the patient gets better. Mood improves, fear abates, optimism returns. Life is worth living again. In fact, it becomes infinitely more precious because it has had to be fought for.

There is a saying, 'the secret of good health is to have a serious disease and cure it.' Arterial disease may not be completely curable, but it is controllable and doctors who work in chelation and other clinics for the circulation seem to have re-acquainted themselves with the original medical values of 'will this treatment *serve* the patient? not 'will this treatment *suit* the patient?'

Surgery, regrettably, because of its life-draining effect on body reserves, both physical and psychological, to say nothing of financial (either on account of surgery or on account of recuperation afterwards), does not empower the patient. One, two or three bypasses and you can have no more – you run out of spare parts and you run out of physical reserves to take the strain of the operation. Arteries which are cleaned out as in angioplasty can be damaged by the procedure – and it is damaged arteries that cause atherosclerosis in the first place. Plaque has been seen to gather around the heart where the surgeon's sutures position the bypass. Options close in on such patients.

Time and time again chelation clinicians find people at their doors who have been given up by orthodox medicine which can 'do no more' for them.

There is an awful suspicion that in advising the surgical option sooner and sooner, doctors are consciously or unconsciously choosing a group of patients who will best serve their statistics and last longer with them. This is especially true of private medicine in America (and probably elsewhere) where one critic of the cardiac surgery business has observed that the skill seems to be in getting the patient at the exact moment when surgical intervention will produce the most revenue and the least comeback when it fails – in that intervening decade between disablement and death.

This may sound like a terrible indictment of a profession composed largely of caring, responsible people. But why is it that each and every chelating physician has had to fly in the face of the establishment in order to pursue a treatment which does not harm and usually improves patients? Most of orthodox medicine will not even listen or learn about what they have to offer. All of the chelating physicians have been ostracized reviled, excluded and sometimes persecuted. Since there is no danger to health in what they are doing (EDTA has been licensed as a safe medicine, albeit not for the purposes of treating circulatory diseases), then the reason has to be commercial. (They cannot – or should not – say it is because double blind trials have not been done on EDTA and circulatory disease, because double blind trials were not done before bypass and angioplasty were used to treat circulatory disease.)

Let us look at what might happen to the cardiovascular business were chelation therapy to be admitted to its ranks.

Chelation for the Future

At the very time when cardiology is pricing itself right out of the market ($40,000 dollars for a bypass, £25,000 in the UK – prices are high because of the complexity of the surgery and all the intensive care and equipment which accompanies it), chelation clinics, on the contrary, could be set up very cheaply.

Since the treatment does not require a sterile environment, clinics could be set up in ordinary rooms adjacent to doctor's surgeries, or elsewhere. Forty or fifty outpatients could be treated at a time by one or two doctors at most and possibly the same number of nurses. (It is not labour or surveillance-intensive). All that is needed in the way of equipment is a sphigmomanometer for measuring blood pressure, stands for suspending the drip bags and fifty chairs! Plus supplies of EDTA and inclusions, infusion bags, and a few emergency drugs, etc.

Patients could be treated on two levels: full-scale treatment for those who had full-blown circulatory disease: mini-chelations for those showing early signs of cardiovascular disease, or with a history of the disease in their families.

British Aims with Coronary Heart Disease

This preventive aspect seems of particular value in view of the British Government's determined efforts to reduce coronary heart disease in the UK.

In 1992, a massive nutrition task force was set up funded jointly by the Department of Health and the Ministry of Agriculture, Fisheries and Food, charged with the job of drawing up a plan to meet the dietary targets set out in the Government's 'Health of the Nation' white paper. This worthy aim, besides acknowledging at last the vital part played by diet in maintaining health, is part of an attempt to bring down the rate of death from heart disease and stroke in Britain by 40 per cent by the end of the century, as well as see reductions in obesity and improvements in blood pressure (an early sign of circulatory disease).

How much worthier to consider what would be a parallel and inexpensive pilot study of the preventive and recuperative effects of chelation therapy on heart disease and strokes? But are we as far away from this as we think?

What is Happening in the UK Today?

There seems little doubt that chelation is being at least *considered* by British Health Authorities, individually and jointly, when letters replying to requests for chelation therapy are examined 'between the lines'.

Take for example this excerpt in reply to a request for chelation therapy for case history number four:

The Department [UK National Health Management Executive] has sought to assess the effectiveness of chelation therapy in the treatment of cardiovascular disease, by consulting experts in the relevant field. We have concluded that there is *at present* [my italic] no evidence that it represents a viable treatment for this condition.

A second example from another patient requesting chelation stated that they were not purchasing it *this year* but may be considering it in the future.

However, some patients in the UK have been successful in securing their ECR (extra-contractual referrals) for treatment outside the accepted delineations of the National Health. In 1989 the then Health Minister clearly stated that chelation therapy was available on the National Health. This statement was supported by the existing Health Minister in 1992 with the proviso that a referral was required from a physician sympathetic to the treatment.

Experience has acquainted those who are submitting requests with a subsidiary condition: funds have to be agreed and found as well as permission given. This is the biggest stumbling block to date. But patients from Manchester, Swindon/Marlborough, Lothian, Dorset, Wirral, Hertfordshire, Greenwich/Bexley and Ealing/Hammersmith/Hounslow have been given permission. (NB: Patients who have private insurance are faring no better: in fact, there are more hopeful signs of a breakthrough in the public sector than in the private sector.)

Elsewhere

The contemporary picture is much the same in America as it is in Britain – chelation is practised but is officially unrecognized and is effectively 'on hold'. In America, court cases have been fought in an attempt to get Medicare (the largest health insurance organization) to pay for patients who can no longer be treated by standard medical procedures.

In Canada, the situation is worse. In 1993, the Health Protection Branch of the Federal Health Minister started seizing and turning back all shipments of injectable drugs addressed to physicians who were using them for chelation therapy – this despite the fact that EDTA is a medically approved substance.

Yet Canada is a signatory (as is the USA) to the WHO's 1989 Helsinki Declaration wherein Section II (1) states: 'In the treatment of the sick person the physician must be free to use a new diagnostic and therapeutic measure if in his or her judgement it offers hope of saving life, re-establishing health or alleviating symptoms.'

Patients' Rights

This raises one of the major issues of our time – the rights of patients to choose their own treatments, having been presented with all the alternatives available. In Britain, National Health Policy has stressed this in recent years. In its official publications, the 'Health of the Nation' and the 'Patients' Charter' it has expressed both the wish that GPs respond to the wishes and needs of patients and also the desire that patients take increased reponsibility for their own health.

It sees the provision of health care at the basic, local level as a partnership between patient and doctor, but wants patients to find out more and have more say in their treatment.

This implies the all-important need for knowledge on the part of the patient, plus the power to implement it. That seems to be what is missing now. Leaflet information is readily available about surgical measures to treat cardiovascular disease, but is less readily available about alternative views, such as diet or anti-stress measures. Moreover, leaflets published by heart charities and cardiac information centres tend to, if not exactly trivialize surgical options, at least make light of them. Cartoons are often used to show patients cheerfully contemplating major surgery, with no reference even to medical alternatives, such as drug therapy (now shown to be just as effective as surgery – *see Introduction*).

The more realistic view of Professor Vincent is of value: 'Cardiac surgery is clearly a highly-invasive and very disturbing thing, involving stopping the heart and starting it, and the brain having to be infused. If you take a patient with a good strong heart muscle who is otherwise well, then the chances of surviving surgery are 99 per cent. If you take a patient who's got a poor heart function who may be unwell, then the risk might be 10 per cent mortality. It's quite low: we're not talking about 50 per cent risk of dying of serious complications because they simply won't be selected.'

So what happens to the presumably significant proportion of coronary bypass patients who do not have strong enough heart muscles? Are they told about chelation therapy? According to Dr Perry, only 1 per cent of patients come to chelation because they have been referred by their doctor. 'In addition,' says Dr Perry, 'we are largely seeing patients at the end of their treatment situation when their doctors have given them up.' Dr Perry's view is that the situation will not change significantly, however good EDTA is for patients with circulatory problems, until clinical trials are done.

But who will pay for them? As said before, EDTA's patent has expired so no drug company can monopolize it and recoup their expenditure by hugely profitable sales.

There are those who conjecture that drug companies could be blocking the admission of cheap chelation into the fold of circulatory disease. The primary physician is the key lynch pin in deciding what drugs or treatments are to be recommended to the purchasing/consulting public. At a parliamentary committee meeting to discuss chelation in early 1994 in London it was alleged (by Richard Thomas, ex-editor of the *Journal of Alternative & Complementary Medicine* and author of a book on heart disease, *The Natural Way with Heart Disease*, Element Books, London, 1994) that in the UK alone drug companies spend £124,000 per annum on promotion per doctor.

Examining this evidence cannot help but lead, at times, to favouring the latter of the two theories currently on offer as to why EDTA chelation therapy is not accepted, that is, is it a cock-up or is it a conspiracy?

The Orthodox Dilemma

Let us not underestimate the difficulties it would present to modern medicine were the whole edifice of cardiovascular surgery to come tumbling down. (US chelation/vitamin C therapy proponent, Professor Cheraskin of Alabama Medical Centre, quotes the current value of bypass surgery alone in America as $3.5 billion. The total value of the cardiac industry to the US is estimated at $6 billion.)

A Canadian journal puts the dilemma more graphically when it lists the people whose jobs could be threatened: 'cardiac surgeons and theatre staff; life support machine and technical staff; cardiac care units and specially trained personnel; angiographers and other diagnostic staff; makers of technology, such as electronic firms who supply monitoring and diagnostic equipment; aftercare units and their adjuncts, for example, physiotherapists, masseurs and counsellors, etc; specially equipped ambulances and staff; resuscitation staff; teaching posts, research groups; spare parts organizers; blood suppliers...and last, but not least, and quite possibly the sting in the tail, pharmaceutical companies who supply the cardiac industry with drugs.'

In view of classic trials, such as the Veterans, CAST and finally RITA (not yet completed), all of which question in one way or another the advisability of much of heart surgery, is it not incongruous to call for a four-fold increase in heart surgeons to meet this health-care crisis, as has the Joint Cardiology Committee of the Royal Colleges of Britain?

There are some positive signs, however. After decades of alternative therapists insisting that dietary and nutritional measures are the two main weapons we have against all degenerative disease, at last recognition of this is being reflected in small trials and studies receiving funding.

Upward Trends

The government in Britain has decided to increase its support for research into antioxidant nutrients and two new projects are to be funded at the Free Radical Research Group led by one of the world's leading researchers of free radicals, Professor Anthony Diplock.

News from the British Heart Foundation indicates that it is funding a trial at an Oxford hospital to study the effect of garlic on reducing cholesterol levels. And research was begun in Cardiff to investigate the protection against heart disease offered by eating oily fish and fish products.

These kinds of projects may seem more like a breath of fresh air than the actual winds of change, but they are nonetheless steps in the right (preventive) direction.

Advice to Prospective Patients

For those seeking any treatment which is still a novelty there is bound to be difficulty in achieving such ends. However, chelation is practised from within the medical profession and as such pressure can be brought to bear on one's GP to recommend it.

Ozone/oxygen therapy is usually performed by those who practice chelation as it is such a valuable adjunct to it. (*see Useful Addresses*).

ACAM in America controls the protocol of the chelation process and trains chelating physicians. Because of their role they can furnish lists of addresses of chelating physicians from all over the world (some addresses, including theirs, appear in this book).

Advice from doctors who practise chelation concentrates in the main on the practicalities of procuring the treatment. Patients are advised not to insure privately with any of the large, totally health-oriented, insurance companies. It is far better to buy insurance from general insurance companies as they will usually accept the recommendation of individual physicians and not follow usual policy.

Never expect that one course of treatment will cure a disease which has been in progress for most of a lifetime. Circulatory disease is multi-faceted and as such requires more than one approach to bring the body back into homeostasis. Furthermore it requires a transformation of the ways which led to the exacerbation of the disease in the first place.

Cures are miraculous: the case histories bear witness to this, but to expect to be cured overnight from a condition which has been developing for decades is unreasonable.

Patience, in the true sense of the word, is required.

USEFUL ADDRESSES

An abridged list of Chelating Physicians or Clinics featured in the text. (Please send a large SAE for UK or international postal coupons for US).

London, UK: The Arterial Disease Clinic, 57a Wimpole Street, London W1M 7DF. Tel: 0171 486 1095. Fax: 0171 486 3816.

Richmond: The Richmond Clinic, 129 Sheen Rd, Richmond, Surrey TW9 1AY. Tel: 0181 332 6685. Fax: 0181 332 6571.

Southern Counties: Liongate Clinic, 8 Chilston Rd, Tunbridge Wells, Kent TN4 9LT. Tel: 01892 543535. Fax: 01892 545160.

Midlands: The Arterial Disease Clinic, Haseley House, Haseley, Nr Hatton, Warwickshire CV35 7LS.

Netherlands: P. Van Der Schaar, MD, PhD, DIPL, Renheide 2, Leende 5595XJ, Netherlands. Tel: (31) 4959 2232. Fax: (31) 4959 2418.

General List, USA: ACAM (American College for Advancement in Medicine), 23121 Verdugo Drive, Suite 204, Laguna Hills, CA 92653. Tel: (714) 583 7666, (800) 532 3688. Fax: (714) 455 9679. ACAM will provide an updated membership list for referrals (domestic and overseas) by writing to the above addresses. (NB: The USA Chelating network covers 46 states. The International Network covers more than 30 countries, including Argentina, Australia, Bahamas, Belgium, Brazil, Canada, South America, Denmark, Dominican Republic, Egypt, France, Germany, Hong Kong, Hungary, Indonesia, Ireland, Italy, Malaysia, Mexico, Netherlands, Netherlands-Antilles, Norway,

Panama, Philippines, Puerto Rico, Saudi Arabia, Spain, Switzerland, Taiwan (R.O.C.), Venezuela, West Indies (Jamaica).

Research Papers

UK: Send a large SAE to ADC London or Midlands (addresses above).

USA: Send a large SAE to the McDonagh Medical Centre, 2800-A Kendallwood Parkway, Kansas City, MO 64114. Tel: (816) 453 5940. Fax: (816) 453 5940.

Alternative Views/Information about Medical Practices and Drugs

UK: *WDDTY* (What Doctors Don't Tell You) Magazine, 4 Wallace Road, London N1 2PG. Book: *Dirty Medicine* by Martin Walker, Slingshot Publications, BM Box 8314, London WC1N 3XX.

USA: *Dr Julian Whitaker's Health and Healing Magazine*, 7811 Montrose Road, Potomac, MD 20854. Book: *Racketeering in Medicine* by James P. Carter, MD, Hampton Roads Publishers, USA, 1992.

Oxygen/Ozone Therapists

UK: All chelating physicians mentioned above do a form of oxygen therapy. For general information about its availability in the UK, send a SAE to Echo UK, 13 Albert Road, Retford, Notts DN22 6JD. Tel: 01777 710 292. Fax: 01777 860 737. For further UK network information (representatives in the Channel Islands, Co. Clare, Ireland, Leicester and Manby) write to Derek Wolfe (address below) with a SAE.

The Richmond Clinic in London specializes in ozone therapy. Derek Wolfe ND MRN (London and Devon) specializes in HOT, a form of oxygen and light therapy. His address is: Naturopathic Practice, 'Newton Mill', Newton-St Petrock, Nr Holsworthy, EX22 7LP. Tel: 01409 281454. Fax: 01409 281454.

Germany: HOT Ozone Therapy: RM-medico, med.Gerate gmbh., Frankfurter Str. 74, D-64521 Germany. Tel: (49) 6152 7873. Fax: (49) 6152 84653.

Ozone Therapy: Siegfried Kamper, Arbeitskreis f. Ozontherapie, Grothusstr 10, Germany. Tel: (49) 209 469369. Fax: (49) 209 42546.

Nutrition (Societies)

SPNT (Society for the Promotion of Nutritional Therapy), First Floor, The Enterprise Centre, Station Parade, Eastbourne BN21 1BE. Tel: 01323 430 203. Fax: 01323 430 516.

BSAEM with BSNM (British Society for Allergy and Environmental Medicine with British Society for Nutritional Medicine), Administrative Secretary, Acorns, Romsey Road, Cadnam, Southampton SO4 2NM. Tel: 01703 812124.

The Nutrition Society, 10 Cambridge Court, Shepherd's Bush, London W12. Tel: 0171 602 0228.

ION (Institute of Optimum Nutrition) Blades Court, Deodar Road, London SW15 2NU. Tel: 0181 877 9993. Fax: 0181 877 9980. (Mentioned in Chapter 7, page 112).

Dr Stephen Davies, The Stone House, 9 Weymouth Street, London W1N 6HQ. Tel: 0171 580 3526.

HRT (Hormone Replacement Therapy), Amarant Trust, 56-60 St John Street, London EC1M 4DT. Tel: 0171 490 1644.

TM (Transcendental Meditation Network) Freepost, London SW1P 4YY.

Bibliography

Brecher, H & Brecher, A. *Forty Something Forever*, Healthsavers Press, USA, 1992.

Brown, R. *Conquering Heart and Artery Disease*, ADC, UK, 1990.

Gordon, F., MD (*see* Walker, M., DPM.)

Halstead, Bruce W., MD. *The Scientific Basis of Chelation Therapy*, Golden Quill Publishers, Inc., USA, 1979.

Holford, P. *Super Nutrition for a Healthy Heart*, ION Press, London, 1989.

McCabe, Ed, *Oxygen Therapies: A New Approach to Disease*, Echo, 13 Albert Road, Retford, Notts. DN22 6JD.

McDonagh, Dr E. W. *Chelation Can Cure*, Platinum Pen Publishers, Inc., USA, 1983, 1992.

Walker, M., DPM & Gordon, F., MD *The Chelation Answer*, M. Evans & Co Inc., USA, 1982.

Walker, M. and Trowbridge, P. *The Healing Powers of Chelation Therapy* (2nd edition 1990).

Oxygen Therapy

Douglass, Dr Wm Campbell M. D. *Into the Light*, Second Opinion Publishing Inc., Suite 100, 1350 Counter Drive, Dunwoody, Georgia 30338 USA.

INDEX